# SOCIAL WORK PRACTICE WITH PEOPLE WITH DEMENTIA

T0386483

*Social Work Practice with People with Dementia* critically discusses the cultural and discursive contexts in which social work with dementia takes place.

This is because how we think about dementia influences how we treat people living with the condition. The book also explains the demographic context that has made dementia a global public health priority in recent years. The different forms of dementia are discussed in a way that is accessible to a non-medical readership. The book discusses the different settings and circumstances in which social work with people with dementia and their carers takes place and examines the chief elements of the social work role. In doing this, it explains the professional knowledge, skills and values that social workers need in order to practice effectively in this area of growing importance. Part of this is appreciating how approaches to dementia care have evolved over time. In this context, the book discusses how the dominant bio-medical model has been challenged by person-centred and rights-based approaches. As a key part of social work is to offer people choices, the book provides information about a wide range of health, social care and other services that are available, whilst also highlighting the gaps that exist for different groups and in different areas. Case studies and activities help the reader apply theory to practice.

*Social Work Practice with People with Dementia* will be of particular interest to social work students and early career social workers, primarily in a UK context. However, it contains much relevant information about dementia and dementia practice for anyone involved with adult health and social care both in the UK and around the world.

**Peter Scourfield** is a Visiting Fellow in Social Work at Anglia Ruskin University, UK. He is the author of *Using Advocacy in Social Work Practice: A Guide for Students and Professionals* (Routledge).

# Student Social Work

www.routledge.com/Student-Social-Work/book-series/SSW

This exciting new textbook series is ideal for all students studying to be qualified social workers, whether at undergraduate or masters level. Covering key elements of the social work curriculum, the books are accessible, interactive and thought-provoking.

## New titles

**Counselling Skills for Social Workers**
*Hilda Loughran*

**Social Work and Integrated Care**
*Robin Miller*

**Communication and Interviewing Skills for Practice in Social Work, Counselling and the Health Professions**
*Patricia Higham*

**Using Advocacy in Social Work Practice**
A Guide for Students and Professionals
*Peter Scourfield*

**Becoming a Social Worker, 3rd ed.**
*Viviene E. Cree*

**Mental Health Social Work in Context, 3rd ed.**
*Nick Gould*

**Social Work Practice with People with Dementia**
*Peter Scourfield*

# SOCIAL WORK PRACTICE WITH PEOPLE WITH DEMENTIA

*Peter Scourfield*

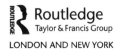

Routledge
Taylor & Francis Group

LONDON AND NEW YORK

Cover credit: © Getty Images

First published 2023
by Routledge
4 Park Square, Milton Park, Abingdon, Oxon OX14 4RN

and by Routledge
605 Third Avenue, New York, NY 10158

*Routledge is an imprint of the Taylor & Francis Group, an informa business*

© 2023 Peter Scourfield

*British Library Cataloguing-in-Publication Data*
A catalogue record for this book is available from the British Library

*Library of Congress Cataloging-in-Publication Data*
A catalog record for this book has been requested

ISBN: 978-1-032-04368-5 (hbk)
ISBN: 978-1-032-04366-1 (pbk)
ISBN: 978-1-003-19166-7 (ebk)

DOI: 10.4324/9781003191667

Typeset in Bembo
by Apex CoVantage, LLC

# CONTENTS

# FIGURES

# BOXES

# INTRODUCTION

In recent years, the growing number of people living with different forms of dementia around the world has come to be recognised as a global public health challenge. According to the World Health Organisation (2017):

> Dementia is a major cause of disability and dependency among older adults worldwide, affecting memory, cognitive abilities, and behavior, ultimately interfering with one's ability to perform daily activities. The impact of dementia is not only significant in financial terms, but also represents substantial human costs to countries, societies, families and individuals.
>
> *(Foreword to Global Action Plan on the Public Health Response to Dementia)*

The Global Action Plan's action areas include raising awareness about dementia; reducing risk; improving diagnosis; treatment; care and support; supporting carers and developing dementia research and innovation. Incorporated within these action areas is the commitment to promote the human rights of people with dementia, to reduce the stigmatisation and discrimination associated with dementia and to produce inclusive and accessible community environments for people with dementia. Many countries around the world, including those of the UK, have developed national dementia strategies whose goals correspond closely to those outlined in the Global Action Plan. Achieving these goals effectively is not just a question of better medical science or of better public services, there needs to be fundamental attitudinal and cultural change for societies and communities to become more inclusive and dementia-friendly.

In the context of this much broader, global agenda, the fact is that many people with dementia require social work and social care services. Therefore, this book has been written in the hope that it can make a modest contribution towards helping social workers to improve the lives of people with dementia, their carers and

DOI: 10.4324/9781003191667-1

families in different ways. Although it is primarily aimed at student social workers and social workers practising in the UK, much of its content should be relevant both to other professions and to an international audience.

It is an assumption of the book that how we think and feel about dementia affects how we interact, communicate and practise social work with people living with dementia. Chapter 1, therefore, invites the reader to reflect critically upon the thoughts and feelings they have about dementia and to examine where such ideas and knowledge about the disease come from. The chapter provides current definitions but also traces how different dementia discourses have developed over time and across different cultures. Historically, dementia discourses have tended to both stigmatise and 'other' those living with the disease, constructing them, at times, as a burden or as tragic cases 'suffering', like 'zombies', a living death. It is argued that, currently, the bio-medical discourse dominates in how dementia is talked and thought about. However, this approach can often tend to focus on organic abnormalities in the brain and, as a consequence, risks failing to see the 'whole person' living with the disease. Therefore, the chapter explains how other more humanising, person-centred and rights-based dementia discourses have taken hold in more recent years. The discussion highlights the importance of paying attention to the imagery associated with dementia and, in particular, the language used in talking about it. Some suggestions are given as to what language to avoid and on appropriate terminology to use when talking to people with dementia and talking about them to others.

Dementia is an umbrella term for many types of neurodegenerative disease and it is important for social workers to have an understanding of the different types of dementia they might come across in their practice. Therefore, Chapter 2 explains the different types of dementia that commonly affect people, outlines their main characteristics and the issues they create for people. It discusses some of the risk factors associated with each type of dementia. The chapter also highlights the fact that, as people age, they are more likely to experience multiple morbidities. Consequently, social workers come into contact with people who are not just living with dementia but also living with other illnesses and disabilities. This makes the social work role more complex and underlines the need for close collaboration with health colleagues and other professionals.

Social work practice with people living with dementia not only takes place within an organisational context but within a broader set of contexts at the national and global level. Understanding these contexts and how they overlap and interact is important because they affect and shape the nature of social work practice. Consequently, Chapter 3 sets out the demographic, social, financial, legislative and policy contexts in which social work practice with dementia takes place. It explains how and why dementia has risen up the global public health agenda. It discusses how, within the UK, national governments have launched their own dementia strategies. Chapter 3 also explains the legislative framework in which social work with dementia takes place. Apart from the Care Act 2014, which applies in England and Wales, social work practice is informed by legislation on mental capacity, mental health and human rights and related policy guidance, for example, on safeguarding.

Approaches to dementia care have evolved considerably over the years and continue to evolve. As with most health conditions, the power of the medical profession and the status accorded to medical science means that the bio-medical model of dementia care is dominant. As noted earlier, this is an approach that primarily focuses on understanding and treating abnormalities in the brains of people with dementia. Although a cure has not yet been found, various drugs and other treatments have been developed to mitigate the symptoms of dementia. However, in the UK, and around the world, partly in response to the bio-medical model, models of person-centred dementia care have developed since the 1980s and 1990s. In the UK, the work of people like Tom Kitwood and his associates has played a huge part in this development. These approaches are more about caring for the whole person and understanding and responding to the individual's feelings and lived experience of the disease. Chapter 4 explains more about these and other approaches to dementia care. For example, in developing his ideas about person-centred care Kitwood wrote about concepts of personhood, malign social psychology and dementia care mapping (DCM). These concepts and their relevance to dementia care are discussed. Since Kitwood, more rights-based approaches to dementia have emerged. To some extent, this has been about ensuring that people with dementia are not marginalised and retain their rights and entitlements both as human beings and as full citizens in society. Therefore, providing an appropriate social and caring environment for people with dementia requires attention to many factors. Many would agree that central to this goal is the need to combat 'dementia-ism' in society. The chapter defines what this is and what needs to happen in terms of attitudinal change in order to enable society to be more dementia-friendly and less stigmatising of people with dementia. Chapter 4 concludes by looking at the role that palliative care and advance care planning (ACP) can play in improving the lives of people with dementia and their family carers.

Whilst the first four chapters of the book are mainly concerned with putting dementia into context, explaining more about the disease and discussing models of care, Chapter 5 focuses specifically on the knowledge, values and skills needed to practise the social work role with people living with dementia. It begins by outlining the main settings in which social work with dementia takes place, highlighting certain challenges facing social workers in the practice environment. The next section discusses the key skills needed, which include empathy, communication and assessment skills including skills in assessing and managing risk. Working with and supporting family carers and informal caregivers is a huge part of the social work role with dementia and several potential stress factors for carers are discussed, together with practice tips on how to manage them. Finally, to practise social work effectively, social workers need to be able to apply life course theories and theories of loss where appropriate. This is particularly true in respect of social work practice with people living with dementia and their carers, whose lives can often be changing significantly whilst experiencing multiple losses. In this context, it is proposed that understanding the concept of ambiguous loss helps to provide a useful insight into what a person with dementia and those around them might be experiencing and how they might be feeling as the disease takes hold.

Key messages of the book are that social work practice with people with dementia should be person-centred, rights-based, inclusive and promote wellbeing and quality of life. Therefore, in order to provide a service that meets these criteria, amongst other things, social workers need to be aware of the range of suitable services that are available to a particular individual and their carers, especially as their needs will change over time. Social workers need to know how to refer to and access these services and, where relevant, they need to know what the costs and eligibility criteria are. Empowering practice means that people should be in control of how their care is delivered and have a choice of services. These can be services provided by the statutory sector but also by private and voluntary organisations. Empowering practice also requires that people are made aware of their rights to services and other entitlements. Choice of services can only be offered and rights to entitlement upheld if social workers ensure that the people with whom they are working have the correct information and knowledge about services. With these points in mind, Chapter 6 aims to outline a diverse range of services that can benefit someone with dementia and those who care for them. It starts by discussing the main health services available and how they are organised and accessed. The next section focuses on social care services and raises some issues about the costs, quality, availability and accessibility of many social care services that need to be taken into account.

Technology-enabled care, in its many different forms, is an area of service which is always evolving. The possibilities of developments in this area for supporting people with dementia are discussed in terms of how they can enhance independence and also provide better peace of mind for families. However, consideration is given to the potential disadvantages of online and technology-enabled care and support services. Technology should be seen as a compliment rather than as a substitute for face-to-face interactions.

Whilst diverse health and social care services are very important for the wellbeing and quality of life of people living with dementia, other services and activities can also be of immense benefit in improving someone's quality of life and providing support for informal carers. A selection of these, including creative activities such as singing, Dementia cafés and advocacy services are discussed. Unfortunately, there are gaps in provision for many potentially useful services, especially in rural areas and in regard to services that are designed around the needs of specific minority groups. Another issue highlighted in this chapter is the low take-up of services amongst certain groups. These are issues that require a whole system approach but social workers can go some way towards addressing them both in their own practice and, collectively, as a profession.

The last part of Chapter 6 highlights developments outside of the UK, and whilst much of the focus of this book is on social work practice in the UK, especially England, this highlights that responding to the ever-growing numbers of people living with dementia is a global challenge. For social workers, the challenge is as much about combating stigma, changing attitudes and promoting rights and social justice as much as it is about providing person-centred care and support. Hopefully, this textbook can make a contribution to going some way to achieving all of these goals.

# 1

# THINKING ABOUT DEMENTIA

By the end of this chapter, you should have an understanding of:

*   Common ideas and myths about dementia.
*   Common definitions of dementia.
*   Your own thoughts and feelings and ideas about dementia and where these originate.
*   Representations and constructions of dementia in everyday and professional discourses.
*   How the way people think and feel about dementia affects their attitudes to people living with dementia, which, in turn, affects the ways in which they interact with them.
*   The appropriate language to use when thinking about and interacting with people living with dementia.

## Thinking and feeling about dementia

It is assumed in this chapter that readers will not be coming to the subject of dementia in a completely 'neutral' frame of mind. Readers are almost certain to have some pre-existing ideas of what dementia is. They are, as a consequence, almost certain to have their own thoughts and feelings about dementia. An interesting question is where do those ideas and feelings come from? Our understanding of, feelings about and attitudes to a subject like dementia are shaped by a mixture of things. As well as the social, cultural and discursive contexts in which we live, the mixture will include our own personal and professional experiences and, where relevant, previous education and training. How we know, understand, think and feel about dementia will inevitably influence how we behave when we meet situations that involve some form of dementia (Sabat, 2001; Downs, Clare and

DOI: 10.4324/9781003191667-2

Mackenzie, 2006). It is therefore a useful starting point to first examine the state of our own knowledge, to consider where this knowledge comes from and, equally importantly, what thoughts and feelings we have about dementia.

## Activity 1.1

1   What would you say dementia is?
2   Where does your current knowledge about dementia come from?
3   What are your feelings about dementia? Give reasons.

Obviously different people will have different responses to all three questions, and, if possible, it would be interesting to share your responses with others. The more responses are shared it would probably become apparent that, whilst it might be possible to arrive at a broadly acceptable definition of dementia, our own experiences of dementia and sources of knowledge about it vary considerably, as will our feelings about it. In common with professional social work more generally, learning about how to practise social work with people living with dementia requires us to be able to reflect critically about what prior knowledge, preconceptions and, possibly unrecognised, prejudices and feelings we are bringing to such study and therefore to our practice (Mantell and Scragg, 2019; Thompson and Thompson, 2018).

Around the year 2000, a nursing colleague shared with me the reviews that he had received from a research paper that he had submitted for publication in a peer-reviewed nursing journal. The subject was a discussion of the positive role that hope could play in the nursing care of people with Alzheimer's disease. My colleague's paper was in a tradition, gaining popularity at that time, of studying the effect that promoting 'hope' can have across a range of nursing situations with chronically ill patients and their carers (Cutcliffe and Herth, 2002). Of the two anonymous reviews received, one was broadly supportive of the paper's publication, believing that it could make a valuable contribution to dementia care. The other reviewer said, in terms, that, from their personal experience, Alzheimer's was a dehumanizing and soul-destroying disease that gradually and eventually robs the sufferer of everything that makes them who they were. In recommending that the paper not be published, they added that, until a reliable cure was found, it was a preposterous waste of time talking about such vague ideas as 'hope'.

I include this anecdote because it made a powerful impact on me at the time and still does. It not only illustrated graphically the strong emotional effect that a form of dementia like Alzheimer's disease can have on those who are close to it, but it also illustrated how someone's personal experiences inevitably shape their outlook on a particular subject. In this instance, the knowledge about Alzheimer's gained from the reviewer's personal experience was elevated above the knowledge expressed in a body of academic literature or research studies. Whether it affected their practice as a practitioner or teacher is unknown. However, it can be assumed that it probably must have in some way. The point of the anecdote is that a subject like dementia has emotional resonance for most people, often based on their experiences and prior knowledge from different sources, sometimes even if that knowledge is second or third hand. It is therefore a complex and often difficult subject. It is useful to try to identify how we 'know' what we do about dementia and also why we have the attitudes we have towards it, in order that we can keep an open mind, maintain a sense of perspective and practise with the appropriate professional detachment. As always in social work, a commitment to reflective practice is essential in this respect (Mantell and Scragg, 2019; Thompson and Thompson, 2018).

## Defining dementia

It is commonly stated that dementia is best described as an 'umbrella term' referring to different conditions that affect the brain and which get progressively worse over time (SCIE, n.d.). As the National Health Service (NHS) website says:

> Dementia is not a single illness, but a group of symptoms caused by damage to the brain.

It further explains that:

> Dementia is not a disease itself. It's a collection of symptoms that result from damage to the brain caused by different diseases, such as Alzheimer's. These symptoms vary according to the part of the brain that is damaged. NHS website.
> *(www.nhs.uk/conditions/dementia)*

The Alzheimer's Society explains:

> Dementia is the name for a set of symptoms that includes memory loss and difficulties with thinking, problem-solving or language. Dementia develops when the brain is damaged by diseases, including Alzheimer's disease.
> *(www.alzheimers.org.uk)*

Using a slightly different emphasis, Stephan and Brayne (2014) state that:

> The term 'dementia' defines a group of syndromes characterized by progressive decline in cognition of sufficient severity to interfere with social and/or occupational functioning, often associated with increasing age.
> *(p. 4)*

There are other definitions of dementia in circulation, all broadly similar, but these can be used as a useful starting off point. Dementia should therefore not be regarded as a single disease or illness. It refers to a range of conditions and syndromes where brain functions are lost and where there is an ongoing decline in different cognitive abilities. In medical terms, it would be defined as 'neurodegenerative', which is a way of saying that the brain cells die or stop working, leading to the various functions controlled by the brain – cognition, memory, motor and social skills and so on – becoming lost or impaired in some way.

Some people use the term dementia and Alzheimer's disease interchangeably or believe that Alzheimer's disease is the medical name for dementia. As the definitions make clear and as will be covered in more depth in Chapter 2, Alzheimer's is a specific disease that damages the brain, but it is only one cause of dementia. The other point to make is that dementia is often used interchangeably with the term 'senile dementia' or often just 'senile' (referring to old age). However, dementia should not be automatically associated with ageing or old age as young people can develop different forms of dementia. Some mental decline happens as we grow older, but the more severe signs and symptoms outlined in the quoted definitions are not an inevitable part of the normal ageing process.

## Early origins of the term

The term dementia itself derives from the Latin *demens* or *de mentia* (which literally means being out of one's mind) and has actually been in circulation with that broad meaning for centuries. For many centuries, disorders like dementia have been seen variously as a sign of possession either by demons or other spirits, as the result of some curse or as a punishment from God for having sinned. Responses, therefore, were either to try to exorcise the demons from the 'victim' by beating them or through other methods or else place the person under restraint for their own good and for the good of others (Porter, 2003). The term dementia became evident in medical discourse from the beginning of the 19th century. The first specific reference to dementia as a mental illness was in a psychiatry text by the French physician Phillipe Pinel (Lyman, 1989). During the 19th century, the most common approach towards 'treating' mental illness in the United Kingdom was through confinement and segregation in asylums (Porter, 2003). At this time, 'dementia', along with 'idiocy', 'mania' and 'melancholia' was a common 'diagnosis' for admission to a mental asylum. Mental asylums varied in their approach. Some doctors, such as Pinel and the Quaker philanthropist William Tuke in England, were pioneering 'moral treatment' and a policy of non-restraint. However, throughout most of the 18th and 19th centuries, people regarded as seriously demented could expect to be placed in some form of confinement and restrained using straitjackets, chains or other physically restrictive measures for their own safety and for the safety of staff and other inmates (Porter, 2003).

## Echoes of the past in the present

As stated earlier, our understanding of and thoughts and feelings about dementia probably derive from a range of sources and experiences – some more obvious to us than others. In Britain today, and around the world, 'dementia', like cancer, is a word that currently has a lot of emotional charge to it and many negative connotations. Whilst this might be related to personal experiences, certain representations of dementia are so deeply rooted and powerful that they live long in the collective memory. Disturbing and graphic images from the history of people labelled as demented being incarcerated and placed in physical restraints are hard to eradicate completely. Such depictions can be seen today in art galleries. It is not unreasonable to suggest that, fuelled by certain representations in the media, historic attitudes towards dementia continue to have a lingering influence, at some level, towards how we approach the topic of dementia today. To some extent, it might be related to the very term 'dementia' itself. Its pre-modern origins and the crude, generalising and damning way in which it was used to label people in the past, have prompted some to argue that we should stop using it as a label today (Corner, 2017). However, the fact is the term continues to be in wide circulation, including official policy documents and medical texts. This will no doubt continue, despite the historical baggage it carries, until something more appropriate is found to replace it. However, the language in which we talk about dementia is important and this will be discussed in more detail later in the chapter.

Many studies have emerged which have analysed how dementia has been socially constructed in different ways over the years (e.g. Harding and Palfrey, 1997). From these, it is apparent that the images, tropes and associations that have been variously used to characterise and construct dementia have deep historical, social, cultural and psychological roots and have almost always been negative. Examining the language and imagery used around dementia reveals a lot about both our attitudes towards and fears about dementia and the people who are living with it. Deconstructing dementia discourses is therefore useful because it can help us better understand the social, emotional and psychological reactions that dementia provokes both in us and others.

## Stigma

The ways that dementia has been represented in different discourses have both reflected and reinforced negative attitudes and feelings about dementia and, as a consequence, stigmatised the people living with it. Here, stigma is taken to mean the 'process whereby certain individuals and groups are unjustifiably rendered shameful, excluded and discriminated against' (Benbow and Jolley, 2012: 165). It also refers to the process whereby someone with dementia feels 'shame about themselves; that they are 'less of a person' because of the symptoms of dementia' (Swaffer, 2014: 709). This process is often referred to as self- or internalised stigma. So there are external and internal dimensions to the stigmatisation of dementia that are interconnected. If we are treated in a negative way by others, with, for example, disgust or pity, then this will most probably have a negative impact on the way in which we see ourselves and damage our sense of self-worth. This process whereby we internalise stigma leads to what Goffman (1963) called a 'spoiled identity'. Fletcher (2019) makes an interesting distinction between 'enacted stigma' and 'felt stigma' in regard to dementia. 'Enacted' refers to the stigmatising behaviours of others. 'Felt' refers to actual experiences of being stigmatised. People need not feel stigmatised by living with dementia even if in wider society negative stereotypes abound. In this respect, Fletcher cautions against the seeming paradox of 'benevolent othering'. This, he argues, can occur when public campaigns that aim to destigmatise dementia by highlighting all the negative ways in which it is portrayed, might actually make those people with a dementia diagnosis feel worse than if the connections had not been made so public. He says that 'ultimately, we should be alert to the danger of accidentally perpetuating that which we seek to challenge' (p. 7). By that token, it could be argued that articles that critique constructions of people living with dementia as if they are 'zombies' do the same thing. The critique inadvertently focuses attention on dementia in a way that makes the possibility of felt stigma even worse. This illustrates the complexity not only about knowing what stigmatises but also in thinking about how to counteract stigma without creating unwanted consequences.

## Depictions of dementia in contemporary popular culture

Popular culture encompasses a multitude of social activities and practices and is expressed through a variety of different media. It includes TV, radio, cinema, videos, advertisements, leisure, fashion, music, social media and linguistic practices. It refers to artistic and creative activities that are produced by and aimed at ordinary people in all their diversity and construct, reproduce and embody the broadly shared meanings of a particular social system. Popular culture has a powerful effect in shaping our attitudes, tastes and other social practices including, for example, how we interact and speak to each other. Popular culture exerts this influence in a variety of ways – some quite directly and others more subtly, even in a hidden or disguised way. How we are affected by popular culture is a complex process but, by its nature, it is hard for any of us to escape its influence completely (Fiske, 2010). Therefore, how dementia has been represented in popular culture inevitably has some sort of impact on how we understand, think and feel about it.

To illustrate some of the points that have been raised, at the time of writing, there is an ongoing discussion in the British media and elsewhere about whether heading the ball in football is a contributory factor in developing dementia in later life. In December 2020, the *Daily Mail* published an article on this topic online with the headline:

> Tony Dunne asked for a gun to end his torment, Bill Foulkes thought he still played in his 70s and David Herd didn't recognise his own face . . . the 1968 Man United team has been decimated by dementia, here the families tell us their heartbreaking stories.

Expanding on this headline, the article goes on to state that 'Dunne's wife revealed he would hallucinate and ask for a gun to end his torment' and that 'In his 70s, Foulkes thought he still played while Herd began defacing his photos'.

Source: www.dailymail.co.uk/sport/sportsnews/article-9080101/Families-great-Man-Utd-1968-team-decimated-dementia-tell-heartbreaking-stories.html

## Exercise 1.2

1    What impression does this article create about dementia? Give reasons.
2    What sort of emotional reaction does the language used in the article provoke?
3    Apart from articles on this specific topic, can you think of other ways in which dementia is represented in popular culture (e.g. in TV, films or magazine stories) which is either similar or different to the depiction in the Daily Mail article?
4    How do representations of dementia in popular culture impact on the way you think and feel about it?

Each of us will have our own reactions to this story. However, couched in language such as 'torment', 'decimated' and 'heartbreaking', even if you had not heard of the footballers in question, it would be hard not to find it grim and difficult reading on some level. It conjures up a nightmarish view of dementia. It is portrayed as a condition where the 'victims' no longer recognise who they are and would rather kill themselves to escape their 'torment'. Of course, one particular article does not represent everybody's experience of dementia but for a condition that has a long history of negative associations, it provides yet more evocations of dementia as a horrible and dreadful experience. In doing so, it both keeps alive and adds to a long-established narrative and further embeds it in the collective psyche.

In thinking about other depictions, you might have thought of examples that are less graphically nightmarish and more compassionate and sympathetic. For example, the Channel 4 TV series *Great Canal Journeys* featured the actor Timothy West and his actress wife Prunella Scales who was living with Alzheimer's disease whilst it was being filmed. It was sometimes difficult to watch Prunella Scales' mental decline as the series progressed, for the effect on her husband as much as anything. However, the series had many tender, often humorous, moments and showed that a couple in that situation could have a pleasurable experience in each other's company even when one of them has a form of dementia. However, such representations are still relatively rare. Unfortunately, the tropes and wording used in the Daily Mail article are indicative of a depiction of dementia that has become well established and quite pervasive over time.

A study by Low and Purwaningrum (2020) revealed that, in popular culture, dementia is often represented in conjunction with negative stereotyped images of ageing and old age. For example, their research highlighted that:

> The characteristics of ageing portrayed in relation to people with dementia were physical (wrinkles, grey hair, age spots, weakened, frail and vulnerable bodies, physical incapacity), social (retired, inactive, contributing less to society, having less friends), and psychological (living in the past, passivity).
>
> *(p. 9)*

Another common phenomenon found by Low and Purwaningrum is that dementia is frequently equated with Alzheimer's disease and old age, with the media using the terms dementia and Alzheimer's interchangeably or together. This led the authors to conclude that:

> The stereotypical depiction of a person of dementia was of an old person with Alzheimer's disease, who loses their memory, mind and identity, behaves unpredictably and is suffering.
>
> *(p. 12)*

The media therefore mainly utilise the same stock of stereotypes and clichés when representing dementia. This contributes to the stereotyping and homogenising of those who live it.

There is also a possibility that you struggled to come up with many depictions of dementia in popular culture at all. This omission, in itself, is indicative of how dementia remains a taboo subject, best avoided altogether. The invisibility of dementia in much of popular culture sends the message that people living with dementia no longer have a place in the mainstream of society. In this respect, they could be said to be 'socially' dead (Low and Purwaningrum, 2020).

## Dementia as a social death/living death

The concept of 'social death' refers to the phenomenon whereby certain groups of people are considered no longer worthy of social participation and, in other people's minds, deemed to be, for all intents and purposes, 'dead' when they are, in fact, still living. There is much evidence to suggest that people living with dementia come into this category (Brannelly, 2011). A study by Sweeting and Gilhooly (1997) highlighted that going by the way they were perceived and treated by those close to them, many people living with dementia experienced a degree of social death before their biological death. People living with dementia were being written off as 'lost' by their relatives, despite the fact that the people with dementia were not necessarily behaving in ways that contributed to that view. It appeared to be a hard process to resist. Conceptions of dementia as a route into a 'social death' overlap with a similar discourse around dementia (particularly Alzheimer's disease) that see it as a kind of 'living' death, where the body lives on but the 'person' who once inhabited it has died (Gubrium, 1986, 1987; Aquilina and Hughes, 2006). In popular culture, the 'living death' dementia discourse is well established (Peel, 2014). For example, the study by Low and Purwaningrum (2020) found that the media descriptions used for dementia included:

> 'death before death', 'funeral that never ends', 'social death', 'psychological death', 'already dead' 'death that leaves the body behind', 'vegetable', 'there is nobody there', and 'withered shells'.
>
> *(p. 11)*

In popular culture, particularly science-fiction and horror films and books, the expression 'living dead' is a commonly used term used to describe zombies. The product of folk lore and myth, zombies are said to be people who have died and brought back to life as creatures in human form but are brainless automatons unable to think for themselves. They are often shown as relentlessly threatening, attacking and even eating human beings. Zombies are therefore to be feared, which is their chief appeal in horror films and literature. However, it has been argued that discourses that describe dementia as a 'living death' are, unintentionally but unfortunately, referencing the zombie myth (Behuniak, 2011). This runs the risk of constructing people with dementia, on some level, as unhuman creatures to be feared, repelled and kept at a distance because they can harm us. Therefore, the conscious or unconscious use of zombie references in describing dementia, means that we can end up regarding those living with it not just with pity but also disgust, horror and revulsion (Hillman and Latimer, 2017). Whilst such discourses do not set out to do so, the effect is to further stigmatise and even dehumanise people living with dementia (Behuniak, 2011; Hillman and Latimer, 2017).

### War on dementia discourse

Another common dementia discourse uses military imagery to frame the 'war' on dementia (Zeilig, 2013, 2014; Lane, McLachlan and Philip, 2013; George and Whitehouse, 2014; Low and Purwaningrum, 2020). In addition to popular culture, the use of metaphors that talk about 'fighting', 'declaring war on' and 'battling' against dementia can also be found in governmental statements, as well as in communication from charities and other organisations. They are well intentioned and are designed, amongst other things, to demonstrate the resolve to find 'a cure' and the determination not to give in to the damage that dementia causes. However, such war imagery can have the unintended effect of conflating the conditions associated with dementia with the people actually living with dementia, so that they, as well as the disease, become 'the enemy'. This is unfortunate enough, but when unconsciously linked to the zombie discourse it conjures a horrific picture of people with dementia as an army of invading zombies to be both dreaded and repelled.

### Dementia as a burden discourse

In many dementia discourses, the words 'dementia' and 'burden' are often paired together (Low and Purwaningrum, 2020). The burden referred to can sometimes mean the burden of stress faced by personal carers but, often, the burden in question is the financial or economic burden of dementia either for the individual or, more often, society generally. So for example, an editorial article in the *Lancet Neurology* journal published in 2018 had the title 'Response to the Growing Dementia Burden Must Be Faster'. It goes on to state:

> According to 2017 estimates from WHO, nearly 50 million people are living with dementia, and by 2030 the number is expected to reach 82 million. As this figure grows, so too will the need for support and care for people with

dementia, which is projected to cost US$ 2 trillion globally by 2030. The need to prepare for and try to prevent some of this personal and financial burden has received increasing attention, most notably with adoption by the World Health Assembly last year of the WHO global action plan on dementia.

*(Editorial Lancet Neurology, 2018: 651)*

In a similar vein, a report by the Cambridge Alzheimer's Research Trust in 2010, subtitled 'The Economic Burden of Dementia and Associated Research Funding in the United Kingdom' stated:

> The combined health and social care costs of dementia are estimated at £10.3 billion in 2008, compared to £4.5 billion for cancer, £2.7 billion for stroke and £2.3 billion for CHD. Using UK prevalence data, the health and social care cost per person with disease was estimated at £12,521 for dementia, £2,559 for stroke, £2,283 for cancer, and £1,019 for CHD. In terms of societal cost, dementia also posed the greatest economic burden at £23 billion followed by cancer at £12 billion, CHD at £8 billion and stroke at £5 billion.
>
> *(Luengo-Fernandez, Leal and Gray, 2010: 7)*

There are many such reports in circulation and they often get taken up and quoted in the news media and other outlets using the same language. They are making an important point that health and social care costs money and that societies and governments need to prepare to ensure that these costs are met. However, as with other discourses, an unintended consequence of talking about dementia in these terms is to position people living with dementia as a [growing] economic burden on the rest of society. When the economic burden representation of dementia becomes entangled in the public imagination with other common representations of dementia as an 'invading enemy' and as a [silent] 'epidemic' (Peel, 2014), it helps create an artificial distinction between 'us' and 'them'. The implications of this process for people living with dementia being constructed as 'them' in this case can be very significant and damaging.

## People living with dementia constituted as 'the other'

Othering refers to the process whereby an individual or groups of people attribute negative characteristics to other individuals or groups of people that set them apart as representing that which is opposite to them (Teo, 2014). As a consequence, the 'other' group is more easily stigmatised, marginalised and dehumanised. One of the most infamous and extreme examples of othering happening in history is the treatment of Jews in Nazi Germany. However, evidence of 'othering' can be seen more recently in the treatment of certain groups perceived as alien, 'risky' or threatening for different reasons, for example, people living with AID/HIV (Joffe, 1999) or immigrants (Epps and Furman, 2016).

When burden discourse leaches into other common discourses on dementia, it can contribute toward the othering of people living with dementia. This discourse helps to create a damaging division between 'us' and the growing number of 'living dead' (them) threatening to overwhelm 'our' health and social care systems and constituting a drain on society's resources.

## Bio-medical discourse

Within health and social care, the most commonly used discourse with which to understand and talk about dementia is one that derives from the 'bio-medical model' (Parker, 2001). Because it is the way in which health professionals primarily conceptualise dementia, this way of understanding it has filtered into everyday use, including amongst people living with dementia and their carers. Dating back to the work of medical scientists in the 19th century, the bio-medical discourse regards dementia, first and foremost, as a disease of the brain (Adams and Bartlett, 2003; Lyman, 1989). Bio-medical discourse is infused with medical classifications, labels and terminology such as 'neuro-pathological', 'neuro degenerative, 'cerebrovascular', 'fronto-temporal' and so on, which reflects the medical scientific practice of classifying and labelling different conditions and behaviours. It is a sign of how well established and pervasive the bio-medical discourse is that people living with dementia and their carers will often use these terms to describe their condition (Fletcher, 2020). Indeed, non-medics can often feel if they have accomplished something significant by using medical terms such as those mentioned. Unlike the more emotionally charged terminology of 'torment', hell' or 'living dead', there is a feeling of scientific precision about bio-medical language. The dominance of the discourse is such that it would be impossible to write about dementia without using language that is so well established in medical circles and is used throughout the health and social care system. Therefore, for this reason, it should be borne in mind when reading this book that the use of bio-medical terminology does not imply the uncritical acceptance of the bio-medical model of dementia.

As suggested, an advantage of the bio-medical discourse is that it avoids emotionally charged language and aims for clinical objectivity in talking about different forms of dementia. Another advantage is that medical labels can help facilitate access to certain services. Sometimes people and their carers can be reassured by having a medical diagnosis (Parker, 2001). However, at its worst, bio-medical discourse can be very reductive, in that it begins and ends with the brain, and the person (whose brain it is) can get lost in the process. This impression is not helped when bio-medical imagery features in popular discourse. As Low and Purwaningrum (2020) found:

> [the] biomedical frame was often accompanied by digital illustrations of disintegrating heads or brains or neuroimaging scans, which serve to de-personalise the disease and emphasises a reductionist biological viewpoint.
>
> *(p. 10)*

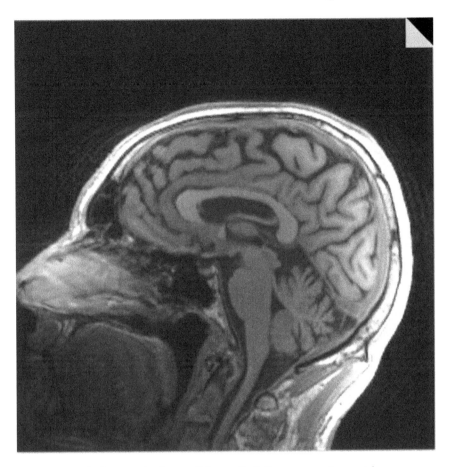

**FIGURE 1.1**    The brain is the focus of bio-medical discourse on dementia[1]

A discourse that primarily focuses on the functions and malfunctions of the brain risks constructing people – all who will have their own individual biographies, situations and feelings – as machines that are malfunctioning because they have a faulty control centre. Figure 1.1 is an MRI scan of my [the author's] brain. I do not think it manages to fully capture the person who I am. In fact, I feel somewhat alienated when looking at it. However, it is this aspect of 'me' that will be the focus of a neurologist's attention. Parker (2001) has argued that:

> A central outcome of the bio-medical approach is that the person becomes subsumed beneath the label. It is the behaviour or the disease that is seen and reacted to rather than the person. The person is 'lost' twice in metaphorical terms – lost as he or she becomes subject to those professionals defining, categorizing and treating their 'condition', and increasingly 'lost' to the pathological changes causing the disease to progress.
>
> *(p. 332)*

Parker not only makes the point that human beings are more than our brains (the vital organ that it is), he also highlights that representations of dementia in popular and medical discourses are linked by the concept of loss.

## Dementia and loss

The different representations and conceptualisations of dementia that have been discussed have emphasised different aspects of dementia. However, whichever way dementia is conceptualised, different representations intersect around the concept of loss. Dementia is associated with experiencing multiple losses (see Chapter 5 for more on theories of loss). These might include loss of memory, loss of sanity, loss of relationships, loss of communication, loss of lifestyle, loss of respect, loss of status; loss of independence, loss of the future, loss of personhood and, perhaps most fundamental of all, loss of self. This would apply not only to the person with dementia but also to those in close relationships with them. Whether a person with dementia is described as having 'lost cognitive function', 'lost their sanity' or 'lost their marbles', it is no surprise that thoughts of dementia can provoke strong feelings of fear, sadness, horror and dread. This possibly explains why, for some, dementia, or certain aspects of it, is a taboo subject altogether.

It might be thought that some of the points made about reactions to dementia in this and preceding sections are fanciful and don't have much purchase in the real world. However, research consistently reveals that stigma is very real and that common attitudes to dementia are often very stereotyped and can include all of the reactions described earlier (Alzheimer's Disease International, 2019). Working to combat the stigmatisation and othering of people living with dementia forms an important part of the social work role and that requires a different mindset and a different linguistic and visual vocabulary.

## Humanising discourses

Low and Purwaningrum (2020) found that 'there were examples of more positive depictions of dementia including expressing love and individual agency and experiencing personal growth (p. 10)' in popular culture, but that these were in the minority. However, there has been a conscious effort in recent years by dementia-friendly communities and dementia enabling organisations to counteract negative stereotypes of dementia in order to combat the stigma associated with it, which have been fuelled and perpetuated by the very discourses reviewed earlier. Often this has been through the active involvement of people living with dementia. Studies show that representing dementia in this way can 'improve positive attitudes and reduce the negative stereotypes associated with living with dementia' (Phillipson et al., 2019: 2680).

The most effective antidotes to the dehumanising and stigmatizing effects of much popular discourse are those depictions that humanise the person living with dementia without denying the struggle it can be to live with it, both for the person themselves and those around them. Positive depictions have to acknowledge the realities of dementia or else they are too easily dismissed as simply as Pollyannaish or a form of wishful thinking propaganda. Accounts that acknowledge the challenges of living with dementia but also manage to preserve the personhood and humanity of the person living with it are few in number but are growing, as the taboos around the topic are gradually chipped away.

A well-known account of living with dementia which is non-medical, 'warts and all', but nevertheless conveys a very human and humanising story is that written by John Bayley in the late 1990s. Bayley was a literary critic who was married to the British Booker Prize winning novelist Iris Murdoch. Still writing novels, Murdoch was diagnosed with Alzheimer's in 1995 whilst in her mid-70s. Bayley, her husband for 43 years, was by her side when she later died in a nursing home in 1999. Bayley wrote a trilogy of memoirs about his life with Iris Murdoch. The first was *Iris: A Memoir* published in 1998, shortly before her death. Those books were later adapted for the cinema in the film *Iris* released in 2001. What emerges is a difficult, often painful account of a relationship affected by Murdoch's condition and the challenges both she and her husband faced as they struggled to cope with it as it progressed. However, whilst Bayley writes candidly about the dark moments in their life together, the tone is not unremittingly negative. In places, it is tender and intimate. The reader never forgets that Murdoch had a non-dementia identity and had a rich and varied life containing many achievements. As the 'old' Iris ebbed away, Bayley describes how they continued to communicate on some level, how she had moods and feelings, how she was capable of expressing her likes and dislikes and how, despite the loss of many social skills, she retained certain social reflexes, such as smiling at a visitor to the house despite not knowing who they were. There were even moments of humour to be found, often in response to trying to cope with the trials and tribulations of everyday life. Since the film *Iris* was released more films have tackled the subject of dementia, with focus on the challenges of living with dementia in ways that humanise rather than just perpetuate the old stereotypes. However, even these more sensitive portrayals can often tend to focus on just one aspect (usually the loss of memory) which can misrepresent the many complexities of living with the condition (Woodhead, 2021).

Earlier, the situation of the actress Prunella Scales was mentioned. She and her husband have actively sought opportunities to talk about what it is like to live with dementia (in her case Alzheimer's disease). The *Great Canal Journey* TV programme was one such example. They were also interviewed about their situation by Age UK which published the interview on their website (Age UK, 2021). The following extract conveys the tone:

Interviewer: Can you work now, Prunella?

Prunella:    Yes, but I have to start learning my lines a lot earlier. It takes me a lot longer to remember things than it did when I was 40. But it is not uncommon at the age of 82 to have memory problems.

| | |
|---|---|
| Timothy: | I think perhaps Pru is being a bit over-optimistic about this. However, there is no reason why she shouldn't still do radio, recitals or voice-overs. |
| Prunella: | In our business, actors like to think they can carry on until they drop. I'd like to die on the eighth curtain call. |

Prunella Scales' comment that 'it is not uncommon at the age of 82 to have memory problems' is a perfectly reasonable point to make. In fact, in dementia studies, it has been argued that dementia and normal ageing should be seen as falling along a continuum rather than dementia being seen as categorically distinct from normal ageing (Huppert, Brayne and O'Connor (1994). However, Timothy West knows there is more to it than that in his wife's case and tactfully but constructively qualifies what she says. Prunella Scales does not demur but makes a humorous reply of her own on the dark subject of her death.

Not all humanising depictions feature or are written by celebrities or public figures. *But Then Something Happened* by Chris Carling (2012) is a detailed, sympathetic account of how both of her parents (Fred and Mary) developed different types of dementia. The book tells their stories and explains what this meant for Fred and Mary's relationship and the impact it had on those around them. This book provides many insights into the problems faced. In common with many other personal accounts of living with dementia, it does not attempt to disguise or minimise the tough challenges involved and the difficult decisions to be made. However, despite that, Fred and Mary shine though as people who have biographies, relationships, thoughts, feelings and a meaningful place in other people's lives.

The work of Sir Terry Pratchett the best-selling science fiction author deserves its own mention. In 2007, Pratchett announced that he had been diagnosed with early-onset Alzheimer's disease. From that point onwards, he became a dementia 'activist'. He made it his goal to campaign and raise money for more research into Alzheimer's disease. However, he was also determined to remain a public figure, to raise awareness of dementia and to promote a debate about what it was like to live with it and what needed to change in response, including the need to permit assisted dying when it was wanted. Aware that, for many people, the taboos around dementia contributed towards their 'social death', Pratchett continued to give interviews in the media in the years leading up to his death in 2015. Pratchett's activism reflects a growing trend of different types of dementia activism amongst people living with dementia in recent years (Bartlett, 2014).

## Activity 1.2: Terry Pratchett

Using online platforms such as YouTube and BBC I-player, locate interviews and other public appearances made by Sir Terry Pratchett after his diagnosis with Alzheimer's disease. For example, he can be seen on Channel 4 News at www.channel4.com/news/terry-pratchett-dies-aged-66-alzheimers. He was also interviewed by the Alzheimer's Society for a short piece called 'Terry Pratchett – Living with dementia' at www.youtube.com/

watch?v=H0HIqfMV2cU and he was also the subject of a BBC TV series 'Terry Pratchett – Living with Alzheimer's'.

Bearing in mind that his is just one account of living with one particular type of dementia, reflect on your reactions to what you have seen. How, if at all, has watching Pratchett speak changed your view of dementia? What else do you want to discover about him as a person and about dementia more generally?

Pratchett tried to take control over his situation rather than be framed or positioned by others' viewpoints. His campaigning activities were about improving dementia awareness and arguing for more money to be spent on research and better services. However, he was also making a statement about the rights of people living with dementia and the need to combat their social exclusion.

Although in the minority in popular discourses, it is possible to find more life-affirming, sympathetic and humanising narratives and discourses. Often they emanate from or revolve around personal stories told by the person themselves or by those close to them. These narratives individualise the person with dementia and present less of a stigmatising and reductivist view of dementia as a consequence. They are still painful to read at times, but by retaining a sense of the person as a human being they can help counteract the dehumanisation and zombification noted in other narratives. Pratchett's activist approach to the subject adds another dimension. It makes the point that, as well as being an individual problem and a medical challenge, dementia is also a political issue. This taps into debates about whether dementia should be regarded primarily as a disease or a disability.

## Discourse of dementia as a disability

Concerted efforts by groups supporting people with different types of dementia have been made in recent years to reframe dementia as a disability (All-Party Parliamentary Group on Dementia (APPG), 2019). This move is based on the United Nations Convention on the Rights of Persons with Disabilities (UNCRPD) which the UK adopted in 2009 and defines people with disabilities as:

> Those who have long-term physical, mental, intellectual or sensory impairments which in interaction with various barriers may hinder their full and effective participation in society on an equal basis with others.
>
> *(UNCRPD, 2006, Article 1)*

There are various motives behind framing dementia as a disability. They include the desire to give people living with dementia the protection of equality legislation, to promote social inclusion, to combat oppression and to protect against the effects of medicalisation – that is to say, becoming labelled and defined by the disease to the exclusion of all else. The All-Party Parliamentary Group on Dementia (2019) stated that:

> The framework for this inquiry is based on the social model of disability, which views people as being disabled primarily by barriers in society, not

by their impairment or difference. The social model, on which the CRPD is founded, suggests that there are a number of factors which create or contribute to the challenges, exclusion and discrimination faced by people with dementia. These factors are the social arrangements, behaviours, norms and practices in wider society. It is these environmental factors and personal attitudes that need to be addressed in order to tackle disability in society, and not the individual impairments related to dementia.

*(p. 12)*

The Mental Health Foundation (2015) makes a persuasive case for the adoption of the social model in respect of people with dementia, arguing that:

The further one travels on the dementia journey the more relevant and meaningful is the social model, as it addresses the increasing risks of marginalisation, isolation and oppression as well as the increasing likelihood of experiencing systemic inequalities, abuse and institutionalisation

*(p. 29)*

However, the desire to include dementia within an unqualified version of the social model of disability has been problematised for a number of reasons and whether dementia will be embraced fully under the disability 'umbrella' remains to be seen (Downs, 2000; Shakespeare, Zeilig and Mittler, 2019). However, adopting the language of disability rights and of the disability movement is important. Because this means that rather than simply seeing dementia as an individual tragedy and as a medical issue it places the focus on the disabling effects of the social and cultural environments in which people with dementia live (Downs, 2000). In taking this direction, there is an obvious overlap with the person-centred approach to dementia care developed by Kitwood (1997) which emphasised the importance of personhood and the threats to personhood from malign social psychology. Kitwood's and other approaches to dementia care will be covered in more depth in Chapter 4. However, it is worth highlighting at this point that the adoption of the social model of disability by some dementia groups and their supporters signalled the need to build upon what Kitwood proposed and incorporate a rights-based and socially inclusive approach to dementia.

## Dementia representations, depictions and discourses: some brief conclusions and pointers for practice

The discussion has reviewed common representations of dementia present in popular culture, as well as those embedded in health and other discourses. Because of the nature of the subject, there are many other variants in circulation (see, for example, Adams and Bartlett, 2003; Parker, 2001). Therefore, the review does not claim to be exhaustive. However, it is evident that much of the imagery attached to dementia in popular culture objectifies people living with dementia and provokes strong, negative feelings such as dread, pity and disgust. The bio-medical framing of dementia continues to play a dominant role. This, too, risks the objectification of people living with dementia for different reasons. There are certain overarching themes that link much dementia imagery – the concept of loss being an enduring and significant one. By its nature, the various influences of popular culture can be deep-rooted, subtle, insidious and also very powerful. Consequently, cultural influences can be hard to detect and their traces hard to shake off completely, however hard we might try. Without being too simplistic or deterministic about it, the point is that if we hold certain ideas about dementia it will probably have implications for our practice of social work with people living with dementia. For example, Adams and Bartlett (2003) make the following point about the implications for the practice of adopting a narrow bio-medical perspective on dementia. They argue that:

> bio-medical discourses create therapeutic nihilism and 'warehousing', in which those with dementia cannot be offered a cure and are stored away in institutions in the hope that a cure may one day appear. The bio-medical discourse that often surrounds chronic confusion therefore constructs the work of health and social care workers as a form of 'body maintenance' in which the person with dementia is merely kept clean, fed and watered.
>
> (p. 7)

It is certainly the case that, in previous decades, that scenario has been played out many times for people diagnosed with different forms of dementia. It would misrepresent the medical and nursing professions to say that they still cling to reductivist bio-medical ideas to the exclusion of all others. Nevertheless, for historical reasons amongst others, the bio-medical discourse continues to play a significant part in shaping how health and social care services are organised and delivered in Britain. However, whether it is to avoid bio-medical reductivism or the reductivism that emanates from any of the other discourses a degree of vigilance is required to ensure that, when hearing that someone has a diagnosis of dementia, our thinking does not follow a pre-programmed course based on stereotyped ideas.

Professional social work embraces an approach to practice that is person-centred, strengths-based, anti-oppressive, inclusive and empowering. An important social work role is to challenge stereotypes and to combat social stigma. However, in order to do this effectively and practise professionally, we need to be aware of the influence of our own cultural and social backgrounds. We need to examine the basis of our own beliefs and be able to bring to the surface attitudes and ideas that might have seeped into our way of thinking about dementia without us being fully aware, if at all. The reason for inviting reflection on your own thoughts and feelings about dementia in Activity 1.1 was as an aid to reflexivity and to critical practice (Thompson and Thompson, 2018). We might not use words such as 'zombie', 'living death', 'hell' or 'torment' in relation to dementia ourselves. However, such images, stereotypes and tropes are very much part of the cultural, social and discursive landscape in which dementia has been constructed over many years.

Research indicates that this discursive context not only contributes towards negative perceptions of dementia amongst the public but that many people living with dementia are prone to self-stigmatise as a consequence of internalizing more widely held negative social attitudes (Trang and Xiaoming, 2020).

Sometimes people who live with dementia are able to manage the effects of negative mainstream dementia narratives by developing their own more positive personal narratives (Beard, Knauss and Moyer, 2009). It comes from trying to look for the positives when they arise and recognizing that, challenging as it may be, living with dementia is 'not all bad, all the time' (p. 234). Beard, Knauss and Moyer (2009) found that by positively reframing their personal situations people living with dementia were able to 'challenge the normative victim-orientation and the social disadvantages of . . . biomedical reductionism' (p. 227). This serves as a reminder that living with dementia needs to be understood primarily as a person's individual, subjective experience rather than it being reduced to a generalised set of issues such as 'cognitive loss', 'organ failure' or 'behavioural problems'.

Positive reframing is about trying to take a more optimistic and balanced perspective rather than seeing life with dementia as one of nothing other than multiple losses and inevitable 'social death'. This strategy might not be possible for all people living with dementia, especially those in the latter stages. However, it demonstrates that it is possible for people living with dementia to disrupt clichéd narratives, resist self-stigma and achieve an empowered identity. Reframing involves challenging negative and outmoded dementia stereotypes and avoiding slipping into discursive practices that either consciously or unconsciously 'other' the person involved. Amongst other things, this involves being mindful of the language we use.

## The importance of language

The language that we use in social work, as in all social relations, is never 'neutral'. It constructs the world rather than simply reflecting or describing it. The meanings contained in language are also not stable. They change over time and according to context. Therefore, social workers need to be aware of the power of language in all aspects of their practice (Gregory and Holloway, 2005). It has already been discussed how some people think that the very word 'dementia' should be abandoned because of its negative associations and its power to stigmatise (Corner, 2017). However, as explained earlier, dementia is a word widely used around the world, not just in popular discourse but also in professional health and social care discourses. Also, because dementia is not a specific illness but an umbrella term for various illnesses and diseases, it has been suggested that retaining the term helps provide a collective identity in the pursuit of disability rights (Adams and Bartlett, 2003). It provides a rallying point for disparate groups of people living with different types of dementia. Whatever our personal feelings about it, the fact is the word dementia cannot simply be expunged. However, we can and should be sensitive in how we use it and its derivatives.

## Activity 1.3

Dementia Australia (2018: 1) make the following statement about the language used in relation to dementia.

> The words used to talk or write about dementia can have a significant impact on how people living with dementia are viewed and treated in our community. The words used in speech and in writing can influence others' mood, self-esteem, and feelings of happiness or depression. A casual misuse of words or the use of words with negative connotations when talking about dementia in everyday conversations can have a profound impact on the person with dementia as well as on their family and friends. It can also influence how others think about dementia and increase the likelihood of a person with dementia experiencing stigma or discrimination. Appropriate language must be:
>
> - Accurate
> - Respectful
> - Inclusive
> - Empowering
> - Non-stigmatising

1 With this in mind, what do you think is the most appropriate language when talking to or about someone who has dementia? What do you think is the least appropriate language? Give reasons in both cases.
2 What language do you think is appropriate and what might be inappropriate when talking about *the impact* of dementia on people living with it? Give reasons.

There are various useful guides to what language to use in relation to dementia. The *Dementia Language Guidelines* cited in Activity 1.3 which come from Australia have been shared around the English-speaking world. For example, the US-based Dementia Action Alliance (2015) used them to produce '*Words Matter: See Me Not My Dementia*'. In the UK, the Dementia Engagement and Empowerment Project (DEEP) published '*Dementia words matter: Guidelines on language about dementia*' in 2014. These organisations have produced these guidelines by involving people living with dementia and those caring for them. Such guidelines can never claim to be definitive and, as highlighted, language can change. However, the guidelines convey the language which was preferred by the people themselves, which is an important basis for any such guide. Currently, the guides are fairly unanimous in explaining that preferred words to use about people with dementia are:

- Person/people with dementia
- Person/people living with dementia
- Person/people living well with dementia

Most of the time in this book the expression 'person living with dementia' is used. Although, at times, for reasons of sentence construction and to avoid too much repetition, this is shortened to 'person with dementia'. Both forms are used because, as the guidelines explain, they emphasise the person first and foremost, rather than their disease. 'Person living well with dementia' is more of a judgement about a specific person's life, so that term is not usually used. According to the guides, words to be avoided include:

- Dementia sufferer
- Victim
- Demented person
- Senile or senile dementia

Words like 'sufferer' and 'victim' are not preferred because they are potentially reductive, making the person an object of pity and therefore they can contribute towards stereotyping. Whilst the word 'dementia' itself is acceptable for the reasons explained earlier, derivatives such as 'dement', 'dementing' or 'demented' are to be avoided, as these are considered negative labels. As explained earlier, descriptions like 'senile' are considered ageist and pejorative. It is always good social work practice to ask people how they identify themselves and take that as a lead. It might well be the case that they choose to use the specific condition they have such as Alzheimer's or Lewy Body. They might say about themselves, for example, 'I am someone with posterior cortical atrophy'. Carers or family relatives might well say that their relative 'suffers from Alzheimer's'. That is their choice, but it needn't be the expression used by the professional. It is not appropriate for social workers to lecture carers or relatives about their language but they can model good practice as a form of education.

DEEP (2014) also says that 'many people with dementia dislike the terms "dementia patient" or "service user" or "client" when these [terms] are used generically to refer to all people with dementia. This is because they imply that they are nothing more than this' (p. 3). Sabat (2001) argues that referring to someone with dementia as 'the patient' (especially when they are not in a health setting) 'positions' them 'malignantly'. It restricts their social persona to just one attribute. Sabat's use of the term malignant in this context is a reference to the phrase 'malignant social psychology' coined by Tom Kitwood (1997). This concept is important in understanding Kitwood's person-centred model of dementia care, which will be discussed in more depth in Chapter 4. Although seemingly more palatable than words like 'sufferer' or 'victim', terms like 'patient' or 'service user' should only be used when talking about people in a health setting or actually using a care service. Even then, they have a homogenizing quality about them. The following quote provides one person's insight into why such terms should be avoided if possible:

> I do not like the term 'patient' unless I am in a hospital or medical setting. If I hear this word used to refer to me in other settings, it weakens me and

I worry I will start acting like a patient and need someone to do even more for me.

*Michael Ellenbogen quoted in See Me Not My Dementia (2015: 5)*

Birt et al. (2017) make the important point that much depends on the individual and what stage they are at in the diagnostic process as to what language is suitable for them. Some people might actively publicly embrace a new identity based on living with dementia – Terry Pratchett is an example. However, others might not be able to acknowledge it and might withdraw from society. This underlines the need to respect the person's agency and take the lead from them.

## Activity 1.4

Later chapters will talk more about the importance of language in social work practice. However, now you might want to consider why people living with dementia and their advocates might object to the use of words such as 'challenging', 'obstructive' or 'difficult' to describe their behaviour. You also might want to reflect on why automatically referring to the spouse or a family member of someone living with dementia as their 'carer' might also be problematic.

This section has highlighted the importance of language in how people living with dementia are both talked to and talked about – how they are constructed. However, placed in the context of the chapter overall, it is worth highlighting that neither dementia nor the people living it are not constructed by language alone. Visual imagery is also important and it has been discussed how, by its use of imagery, the bio-medical approach frame tends to overemphasise the disembodied brain in how it explains dementia. When presented with illustrations such as Figure 1.1, it is easy to forget that, ultimately, it is how the person is affected that matters and not simply the failure of an organ of the body to work properly. Other images can be equally reductive. For example, the DEEP (2014) guidelines highlight how, even when text is trying to present a 'positive image, this can be undone by accompanying it with stereotyped images such as a "fading face or wrinkled hands"' (p. 4). Again, this reduces the individuality of people with dementia by defining them with ageist stereotypes.

## Summary of key points

- Dementia is an 'umbrella' term used to describe a range of progressive neurological disorders. It is not a disease itself. It is a collection of symptoms that result from damage to the brain caused by different diseases.
- How we feel about and understand dementia is inevitably shaped by a mixture of different personal, cultural, historical and social influences.
- Historically, dementia discourses have been negative and have contributed to the stigmatisation and othering of people living with dementia.
- Even today, representations of dementia popular culture still tend to draw on and perpetuate negative stereotypes.

- Much contemporary discourse on dementia is dominated by the bio-medical model.
- In more recent years, discourses on dementia have emerged that are more humanising and are based upon person-centred and rights-based approaches.
- Moves to get dementia accepted as a disability rather than a disease are designed to highlight the disabling effects of social and cultural attitudes. The aim is to promote the equal rights and social inclusion of people living with dementia.
- The way in which frame and think about dementia will inevitably affect how we behave around and practise social work with people living with dementia. This, in turn, has ramifications for their experiences of social work and the social care system more generally.
- Careful consideration needs to be given to the language used when we talk to and talk about people living with dementia. Terms that are reductive and stereotyping such as 'sufferer' should be avoided.

## Note

1  Reproduced courtesy of the Wolfson Brain Imaging Centre – University of Cambridge NIHR BioResource.

## Further reading

Alzheimer's Disease International (2019). *World Alzheimer Report 2019 Attitudes to Dementia*. London: Alzheimer's Disease International.
  This is an important report that takes a global, cross-cultural perspective on attitudes to dementia. It explores the topic of stigma in depth. It has ten expert essays and twenty one case studies from around the world. It also includes nine programmes to reduce stigma.

## *Further viewing*

The personal narratives of living with dementia can be found in the BBC TV series *Dementia and Us* which followed four people with dementia and their families over the course of two years and aired in 2021. Voiced by Dreane Williams, a dementia campaigner who has vascular dementia herself, it provides valuable insights into the impact of living with dementia on people and their families.

# 2
# TYPES OF DEMENTIA

By the end of this chapter, you should have an understanding of:

- The signs, symptoms and causes of common forms of dementia.
- Factors that increase the risk of developing dementia.
- The impact on people living with different forms of dementia.
- The impact on those around people living with these forms of dementia.
- Common medical and non-medical treatments.
- The importance of being aware that people with dementia often have (undiagnosed) comorbidities.
- Some of the rarer types of dementia with which social workers come into contact in their practice.

## Introduction

There are over 100 types of dementia that can affect people (Alzheimer's Society, 2013). Different types of dementia affect people in different ways and different types of support are needed as a consequence. Social workers working with people living with dementia usually work in multi-disciplinary settings. In this context, their medical and health colleagues routinely use bio-medical language and diagnostic labels when talking about the different people with dementia with whom they are involved. Often people living with dementia and their carers find it useful to have a specific medical diagnosis and to understand what that means in terms of the progression and treatment of the disease. Therefore, for these reasons, it is important for social workers not only to know the difference between the different types of dementia but also to be conversant with the relevant medical terminology and have sufficient medical knowledge in order to work effectively as part of a multi-disciplinary team. Thus, although social workers should

DOI: 10.4324/9781003191667-3

be wary of being drawn into a narrow medical model mentality, it is important to be familiar with and to be able to use bio-medical language when appropriate. Chapter 1 highlighted the importance of language in dementia practice and, particularly, the potentially dehumanising effect of constituting people as medical 'cases' through the use of bio-medical language. However, with vigilance, it is perfectly possible to use medical language and still be committed to both the social model of disability and a person-centred approach. Indeed, if social workers want to work effectively with people living with dementia, then they need to pay them the respect of understanding the medical side of their condition as best they can. However, because a little knowledge is always a dangerous thing, the provision of actual medical advice should be left to medically trained colleagues. This is a book aimed at social workers and does not claim to be a medical text. With these caveats in mind, the chapter discusses the most common types of dementia, how they affect both the people concerned and their carers, as well as discusses medical and other interventions that are commonly available. In doing this, some relevant bio-medical terminology is explained. The chapter will also highlight the need for social workers to understand that people living with different forms of dementia will often have other illnesses (co-morbidities) such as hypertension, diabetes, heart problems and depression (Public Health England, 2019a). The potential presence of other health conditions alongside dementia underlines the need for both a full and holistic needs assessment and person-centred care planning when practising social work with people living with dementia.

## Alzheimer's disease

Alzheimer's disease is the most common type of dementia in the UK. It affects more women than men partly because, on average, women are still living longer than men, and the chances of getting Alzheimer's disease increase with age (Alzheimer's Research UK, 2015; NHS, 2021). In the UK, Alzheimer's disease accounts for between 60% and 70% of all dementias (Public Health England, 2019b). However, Alzheimer's does not follow the same pattern of incidence in every country in the world. The incidence of Alzheimer's is much higher in Western Europe, for example, than in Japan and most African countries (Henderson/WHO, 1994; Rizzi, Rosset and Roriz-Cruz, 2014).

## Definitions

The International Classification of Diseases (ICD) which is maintained by the World Health Organisation (WHO) defines 'Dementia in Alzheimer disease' as:

> a primary degenerative cerebral disease of unknown etiology with characteristic neuropathological and neurochemical features. The disorder is usually insidious in onset and develops slowly but steadily over a period of several years.
>
> *(International Classification of Diseases, 2016)*

This definition provides a good opportunity to become more familiar with the medical language often used in conjunction with Alzheimer's disease and dementia more generally.

'Cerebral' in medical terms means pertaining to the 'cerebrum' – the brain. 'Etiology' is a term used in medical science to refer to the causes and origins of diseases. 'Neuropathological' is a medically scientific term that refers to diseases of the nervous system. 'Neurochemical' is the medical term used to describe chemical processes that occur in the nervous system or parts of it. 'Insidious' is a not specific medical term but when used in a medical context means that the illness or disease develops and progresses in an imperceptible manner, often reaching a harmful stage before it is suspected. So, translated, this definition explains that Alzheimer's disease is a disease of the brain and nervous system which (currently) has no known cause and which often slowly 'creeps up' on those who have developed it without them knowing it, at least in the early stages. Stephan and Brayne (2014) explain more about the features of Alzheimer's disease, stating:

> Alzheimer's disease is characterized by a steady and progressive loss of memory and cognitive faculties, including language deterioration, impaired visuospatial skills, poor judgement, and an attitude of indifference. Alzheimer's disease has a distinct neuropathological pattern of amyloid plaques and neurofibrillary tangles predominately in the neocortex, becoming more widespread with disease progression.
>
> *(p. 4)*

Our 'visuospatial skills' enable us to visually identify and process information about 3D objects and also assess the spatial relationships between objects. We need visuospatial skills for many of the activities of everyday life. For example, making a cup of tea requires these skills to be able to identify and assemble the various components in the correct sequence and in the correct place. Someone whose visuospatial skills are impaired would have difficulties using stairs, parking a car or simply recognising objects for what they are. When this happens with someone with Alzheimer's disease, it is known as 'visual agnosia'. The important point to note with visual agnosia is that the person's eyesight is not the problem, it is the brain failing to interpret what the eye sees correctly.

Amyloid plaques and neurofibrillary tangles are deformities of the brain. Autopsies on people with Alzheimer's show that their brains have shrunk significantly more than a normal (i.e. non affected) brain. Post-mortem examinations show that Alzheimer's brain tissue has many fewer nerve cells and synapses (junctions between two nerve cells) than a healthy brain. Apart from excessive shrinkage, examinations of the brains of people who have lived with Alzheimer's disease also reveal 'neurofibrillary tangles'. 'Neurofibrillary' refers to the threads (fibrils) which run through the nerve cells. These 'tangles' are abnormal accumulations of a protein called tau that collect inside the nerve cells. The tangles are dead and dying nerve cells (neurons). Amyloid plaques are abnormal clusters of protein fragments that build up between nerve cells and disrupt cell function.

The cerebral cortex is the outermost layer of the brain, made up primarily of 'grey matter'. The neocortex makes up the largest part of the cerebral cortex and is the centre for higher brain functions, such as perception, decision-making and language. Therefore deformities in the neocortex have an effect on these functions. Alzheimer's disease causes organic damage to many areas of the brain.

Using less medical terminology, the NHS website defines explains that:

> Alzheimer's disease is a progressive condition, which means the symptoms develop gradually over many years and eventually become more severe. It affects multiple brain functions. The first sign of Alzheimer's disease is usually minor memory problems. For example, this could be forgetting about recent conversations or events, and forgetting the names of places and objects. As the condition develops, memory problems become more severe and further symptoms can develop, such as:
>
> - confusion, disorientation and getting lost in familiar places
> - difficulty planning or making decisions
> - problems with speech and language
> - problems moving around without assistance or performing self-care tasks
> - personality changes, such as becoming aggressive, demanding and suspicious of others
> - hallucinations (seeing or hearing things that are not there) and delusions (believing things that are untrue)
> - low mood or anxiety
>
> *Source: www.nhs.uk/conditions/alzheimers-disease/*

## Activity 2.1

From the definitions and descriptions provided, try to imagine what it feels like to be in the first stages of Alzheimer's disease. What sort of things might make you want to get a medical opinion on about what is happening? How might you feel when the doctor informs you that it could be that you have Alzheimer's? What might the reactions of those close to you be?

Check out the Alzheimer's Society YouTube Channel, which, at the time of writing, is located at: www.youtube.com/channel/UC1miDO27ShatLOE4nWAR-YCg Browse the uploaded videos for people talking about their experiences of Alzheimer's. A good example, if you can locate it is: 'Lorraine Brown – my journey with dementia' (www.youtube.com/watch?v=TsV9g8dojkE).

The purpose of the activity is to make sure that Alzheimer's disease is not just understood as neuropathological condition that affects the nerve cells in the brain, it is also an individual lived experience that inevitably prompts a range of emotions.

# Causes

The exact cause of Alzheimer's disease is not yet fully understood. Different theories point to there being a genetic link, but this factor alone does not explain or predict why every person with Alzheimer's disease has it or will get it (Smith, 2004). Currently, there is no effective cure, although symptoms can be controlled and mitigated up to a point through medication and other interventions. Whilst it is not known exactly what causes Alzheimer's to develop, certain risk factors have been identified. These include:

## Age

The likelihood of developing Alzheimer's disease doubles every 5 years after reaching the age of 65. Therefore, the chances of getting it increase with age. That said, it is worth noting that roughly 5% of people with Alzheimer's in the UK are under 65.

## Genetics

The genetic link is complex and not fully understood. However, although the risk might not be that big, a history of Alzheimer's in the family can contribute to the risk of someone developing the disease. The same is true of other types of dementia [see '*Genetics of Dementia*' (Alzheimer's Society, 2016a) for more on this].

## Lifestyle factors

It is suggested that what is good for the heart is good for the brain (see '*The Brain-Heart Connection*' (Global Council on Brain Health, 2020) for more details). Lifestyle factors and conditions associated with increased risk of cardiovascular disease are therefore said to increase the risk of Alzheimer's disease (and other dementias, specifically vascular dementia). These factors include: smoking, obesity, diabetes, high blood pressure and high cholesterol levels. Be clear, these are possible contributory factors and not causes.

## Other risk factors

Other factors have been linked to the development of Alzheimer's disease, such as head injuries, depression and hearing loss, although more research is needed in order to determine what, if any, the linkage is.

*Source: www.nhs.uk/conditions/alzheimers-disease*

## Links between Alzheimer's disease and Down's syndrome

People with Down's syndrome have a higher risk of developing Alzheimer's disease. Autopsy studies show that by age of 40, the brains of almost all people with Down's syndrome show significant levels of beta-amyloid plaques and tau tangles – which are the brain abnormalities strongly associated with Alzheimer's. Statistics from the USA show that roughly 30% of people with Down's syndrome who are in their 50s have Alzheimer's and about 50% of people with Down's syndrome in their 60s have Alzheimer's (Alzheimer's Association, 2021). Not everyone with Down's syndrome develops Alzheimer's symptoms but the risk is higher than in the non-Down's population (NHS, 2021).

## Non-links

At various times, different factors have been linked to Alzheimer's which have turned out to have no scientific basis. Old age in itself is definitely not a factor. Neither is stress, although stressful events might bring a previously hidden dementia condition into the open. It has also been believed that exposure to aluminum or dental fillings causes Alzheimer's, but neither of these beliefs has been supported by research (Cayton, Graham and Warner, 2002; Smith, 2004).

## Diagnosis

There is currently no way of diagnosing Alzheimer's disease with absolute precision. If a general practitioner (GP) suspects that someone might be developing the disease on the basis of the symptoms presented to them, they will do tests in order to eliminate other possible explanations. If there are no obvious alternative explanations, the GP will usually refer to a specialist such as a neurologist or psycho-geriatrician who are often attached to an NHS or privately run memory clinic for further tests. However, there is no simple and reliable diagnostic test for Alzheimer's disease. CAT scans (X-ray imaging of the brain) and MRI scans (magnetic resonance imaging of the brain) are used to identify damage to the brain. Dementia specialists also assess cognitive functioning using mental ability tests. Two commonly used assessment tools are the Mini-Mental State Examination (MMSE) and Mini-Cog test. Although both provide useful screening information, neither could be said to be definitive in determining whether someone has Alzheimer's or not (Arevalo-Rodriguez et al., 2015;Fage et al. 2015, 2019). It has also been highlighted how these tests can have a negative impact on the people taking them. This would not only be in terms of the stress of actually performing in the test but also the lowering of self-concept if someone thinks that they have 'failed' the test. There can also be anxiety about how others' perceptions might change negatively if such a 'failure' occurs (Lyman, 1989).

Mental ability testing can be carried out in someone's own home but is often carried out at a memory clinic. More will be discussed about this service in Chapter 6. The main point to understand is that establishing a reliable diagnosis of Alzheimer's usually takes a range of information to be gathered and assessed over time.

## Activity 2.2 MMSE and Mini-Cog tests

To help you to understand how these tests work and what it is like to do one, you can locate them quite easily online. For example, a version of the MMSE can be retrieved from: www.bgs.org.uk/sites/default/files/content/attachment/2018-07-05/mini-mental_state_exam.pdf and the Mini-Cog from: https://content.highmarkprc.com/Files/EducationManuals/GeriatricResource Binder/mini-cog.pdf

N.B. Do not be tempted to use them in your own practice without specialist training.

## Medication

Readers in the UK should check the latest National Institute for Health and Care Excellence (NICE) guidelines for accurate information on the medication used for all types of dementia. At the time of writing, this can be accessed at 'Dementia: assessment, management and support for people living with dementia and their carers' (NICE, 2018).

## Cholinesterase inhibitors and NMDA receptor antagonists

Cholinesterase inhibitors and NMDA receptor antagonists are two types of drugs used to alleviate or control the symptoms of Alzheimer's disease in the UK (Alzheimer's Society, n.d.). Cholinesterase inhibitors are designed to help common symptoms of Alzheimer's such as memory loss and anxiety. They may also help improve levels of motivation, memory, concentration and thinking. The three drugs currently licensed are Donezepil (Aricept™), Rivastigmine (Exelon™) and Galantamine (Reminyl™). These drugs do not provide a cure and neither are the benefits long term; however, they can slow the course of the illness.

NMDA receptor antagonists work differently from cholinesterase inhibitors. The main receptor antagonist used for Alzheimer's in the UK is Memantine (Exiba™). According to the Alzheimer's Society (2014):

> Memantine is licensed for the treatment of moderate-to-severe Alzheimer's disease. In people in the middle and later stages of the disease, it can slow down the progression of symptoms, including disorientation and difficulties carrying out daily activities. There is some evidence that memantine may also help with symptoms such as delusions, aggression and agitation.
>
> *(p. 4)*

Neither Cholinesterase inhibitors nor NMDA receptor antagonists are said to be addictive but they can have side effects such as nausea, dizziness, headaches and tiredness.

## Other drug treatments

As well as the specific anti-dementia drugs discussed, other forms of medication can be prescribed to help with common effects of living with Alzheimer's (and dementia more generally). For example, because people with dementia are a group with an increased risk of developing depression, they may often be prescribed anti-depressants. It is also quite common for people to be prescribed anxiolytic drugs which are used to reduce the symptoms of anxiety and sleeping problems that can accompany dementia. Antipsychotic drugs such as Risperidone can be prescribed, with caution and often as a last resort, to treat symptoms such as aggression, agitation, restlessness, depressed mood and anxiety, as well as hallucinations and delusions. In the past, unfortunately, it has been the case that antipsychotic drugs have been misused in dementia care, particularly in care homes. The All-Party Parliamentary Group on Dementia (2008) found that over 100,000 people with dementia in care homes were being overprescribed antipsychotic drugs. Since then, medication protocols and better training have been put in place. However, it remains a situation that needs close monitoring.

For a fuller discussion of dementia medication, go to the relevant pages on the NHS website: www.nhs.uk/conditions/dementia/treatment.

## Alzheimer's and polypharmacy

Polypharmacy means taking more than one medicine. As their disease progresses, the chances are that people with Alzheimer's will be taking different types of medication for their condition. They might also be taking medication for other health conditions they have at the same time ('co-morbidities') such as diabetes, hypertension and stroke. If not managed properly, this situation can lead to potentially harmful drug interactions. With more people living longer and with more people developing Alzheimer's and other forms of dementia, it is a growing issue and needs more research (Parsons, 2017). As NICE explains,

> Polypharmacy can be complex to manage, and can sometimes become a problem. When a person takes many medicines, there is a larger risk for side-effects and interactions. The practicalities – taking all your medicines at the right time, and in the right way – becomes harder too.
>
> *(NICE, n.d.)*

Medication is not strictly the professional domain of social workers. However, social workers need to be aware of the potential issues raised by polypharmacy and to be prepared to refer to the person's GP if they suspect the person either is not managing their medication properly or that the various medicines they are taking are possibly interacting in a harmful way. Professionals such as district nurses and care staff can undertake specialised training in medication management and are able to advise on different medication self-management tools such as pill dispensers and dosette boxes. Pharmacists are also a good source of advice about medication and how best to manage multiple medications. It is important to manage polypharmacy properly not just to eliminate or reduce the risk of harm but also to maintain the person's choice and independence by enabling them to be in control of their own medication as much as possible for as long as possible.

## Non-drug treatments

Treatments for different types of dementia that do not involve medication include cognitive stimulation therapy (CST) and cognitive rehabilitation but not cognitive training (NICE, 2018). These are usually carried out by specialist psychologists. There is evidence to suggest that in people with mild to moderate dementia the effects on improving cognition of psychological treatments can be comparable to medical interventions (Spector, Woods and Orrell, 2008). There are other psychosocial treatments for dementia such as reminiscence and life story work that can promote improvements in cognition, mood and communication. However, whilst some benefits have been recorded, the effects of these interventions are said to be 'inconsistent' (Woods et al., 2018). More will be discussed about different nonmedical interventions in Chapter 6.

## The progression and stages of Alzheimer's

The Alzheimer's Society (2021a) explains that:

> Dementia is progressive. This means symptoms may be relatively mild at first but they get worse with time. Dementia affects everyone differently; however it can be helpful to think of dementia progressing in 'three stages'.

Alzheimer's is, indeed, progressive. However, Lyman (1989) cautions against overly deterministic stage attributions to the disease alone. There is no universal 'Alzheimer's sufferer' whose disease can be plotted and predicted through known stages. There will be individual variations in how the disease progresses, not least because of social, environmental and a range of other factors unique to that person. With that said, it is useful to know the broad stages that many people go through so that, if and when they occur, appropriate interventions can be put in place and the person can be properly cared for and supported.

## Early stage

The early stage of dementia is said to last on average about two years. The signs and symptoms that start to emerge during this stage include memory problems, language and communication difficulties, difficulty completing familiar tasks, visual-perceptual difficulties, changes in mood and/or emotion, misplacing things and losing the ability to retrace steps and loss of social confidence often accompanied by withdrawal from work or social activities. These symptoms do not necessarily occur all at the same time and are not the same for everybody. We always need to remember that somebody learning that they have Alzheimer's or any other type of dementia is a unique experience for them and for those close to them. Often, there is bafflement, anxiety and fear about exactly what is happening. Case Study 2.1, which is based on a real-life story, provides some insights into a family's experience of the early stage of Alzheimer's.

## Case Study 2.1: Mary

The narrative is written by Chris Carling, the daughter of Mary and Fred. It is already known that Fred (Mary's husband) was living with vascular dementia. This extract comes from the section of the book titled 'Why didn't we see it coming?'.

> Eventually though Dad insisted he was hanging up his driving gloves. Mum loved going out and still wanted to go shopping so she took to walking over to the Grafton Centre, a shopping mall about ten minutes away from their house by the shortest route which involved crossing a busy road. We used to chat about her outings. From odd remarks I had the impression she was taking a roundabout route.
>
> Concerned for her safety now that Dad stayed at home, I would question her, wanting reassurance she was taking the safest route, the one with the lights-controlled pedestrian crossing over the busy road. But these conversations were always inconclusive. She couldn't tell me in any straightforward way where she went. Her answers were puzzlingly vague.
>
> I realise now that this inability to describe her route was one of the early signs of Mum's dementia. She could get to the Grafton Centre but couldn't say how. And she got there, I eventually figured, taking a longer and more hazardous route – she crossed the busy road where there were no pedestrian lights – because this took her to where Dad used to drop her off and pick her up. It was as though her body knew that way but her mind no longer knew what it was she knew.
>
> Like Dad's anxiety, it was a sign I half noticed in that I was worried and tried to find out the facts, yet I didn't follow through and ask myself: what's going on in Mum's brain such that she can't tell me which way she goes, doesn't remember the names of the streets any more or which of the paths across the common she takes? So long as she managed to get there and back, I put my worries on the back burner. Or was it my head in the sand?

As the year wore on she'd occasionally worry Dad by staying out for hours though she always managed to find her way back in the end. People with Alzheimer's, I later learnt, often get lost in familiar places (Carling, 2012: 189).

## Activity 2.3: Experiences of Alzheimer's disease

The Alzheimer's Society has made a video that features real people talking about what it is like to be told they have dementia, what the signs and symptoms were and what effect it had on their lives. It also includes advice about how to manage the condition in ways that are person-centred. It is called 'The Dementia Guide' and, at the time of writing, it is available at www.youtube.com/watch?v=RLBuygIcttU. Although, over time, the URL might change, it should be easily found by searching for 'The Dementia Guide'.

Reflect on the experience of someone discovering that they probably have Alzheimer's disease. What feelings and thoughts does it evoke? What do you think that people need at this stage?

## Confabulation

In order to try and make coherent sense of gaps in their memories, people living with dementia, especially in the early stages of the disease, compensate through the process of 'confabulation'. Confabulation is more common with Korsakoff's syndrome (discussed later) but is also a feature of Alzheimer's disease in the early to middle stages. According to Brown et al. (2017):

> Confabulation refers to the production or creation of false or erroneous memories without the intent to deceive, sometimes called 'honest lying'. Alternatively, confabulation is a falsification of memory by a person who, believes he or she is genuinely communicating truthful memories. These false memories may consist of exaggerations of actual events, inserting memories of one event into another time or place, recalling an older memory but believing it took place more recently, filling in gaps in memory, or the creation of a new memory of an event that never occurred.
>
> *(p. 1)*

Often, those in contact with people developing Alzheimer's disease misunderstand confabulation, seeing it as the person deliberately exaggerating or making things up. People who confabulate can often be very confident in their memories even after being presented with contradicting evidence. This can create tensions and sometimes conflict especially if they appear to be 'stubbornly' refusing to accept another version of events. When seen in the context of living with dementia, confabulation should be seen as someone trying their best to piece together a coherent story from memories that have become increasingly gappy and fragmented or lost altogether.

## Middle stage

The middle stage of dementia lasts, on average, for about two to four years but can last longer. It is the stage when existing symptoms become noticeably worse, to the point that the person concerned will need more support in managing the activities of daily living, such as using the toilet or preparing food. Memory and thinking, misplacing things, speaking, understanding other people, becoming lost and disorientated in place and levels of confusion are all likely to deteriorate. The person might start having changes in perception by, for example, becoming delusional, paranoid and hallucinating. The middle stage is also when changes in behaviour generally start. These commonly include agitation and restlessness, screaming or shouting, repetitive behaviour, following a carer around (trailing), losing social inhibitions and disturbed sleep patterns. All of these changes will be disturbing and confusing for the person and those around them. It is also common to become depressed in this stage. Carers and relatives will more likely be experiencing increased levels of stress as a consequence. More information and advice can be found on all of these and other symptoms at the Alzheimer's Society, Dementia UK and NHS websites. It is worth highlighting some common issues that either emerge or get worse at this stage.

## Sleep disturbances and 'sundowning'

Of the many changes that people living with Alzheimer's disease experience, problems relating to sleeping are often some of the most noticeable. One of the problems with sleeping for people with Alzheimer's is confusing day and night. Sleep problems are thought to be linked to different factors. For example, the disease damages the brain and changes the way it controls the sense of when to sleep and when to be awake. It might also be linked to the tendency for people with Alzheimer's to take more naps during the day and have trouble falling asleep as a consequence or could be to do with being disorientated due to the inability to separate dreams from reality when sleeping. Related to sleep disturbance is a phenomenon called 'sundowning agitation' or commonly just 'sundowning'. This is where the person with Alzheimer's becomes more agitated and behaves in ways that are even more difficult to understand – more often in the late afternoon or early evening – hence 'sundowning'.

Symptoms of sundowning agitation include disorganised thinking and speech; a variety of motor disturbances including agitation; repetitious physical behaviours; perceptual disturbances such as illusions and hallucinations and emotional disturbances such as anxiety, fear and anger. Help is possible through both medical and psychological treatments but the problems associated with sleep disturbances can be a significant source of stress for family members and carers as well as having a negative impact on the person's and carers' quality of life (McCurry et al., 2000).

## Case Study 2.4:   Else

Else is a 90-year-old woman who has been living with Alzheimer's disease for at least ten years. She lives at home with her husband George who also has mental and physical ill health. They have a live-in carer and their daughter Grete, who lives locally, visits every day. Grete notices that for some time now every day at about 3.00 pm, after a nap, her mother wakes and starts to become more agitated and restless. Even though she has very poor mobility she struggles effortfully to get out of her reclining chair and 'go home' as she says. She is originally from Norway and will often talk in Norwegian about going into Bergen (where she lived as a child) and seeing Alfred (her father). Grete knows that it will pass after about two hours when they have their evening meal. She does not contradict her mother or remind her that she actually is at home and that Alfred is long dead. Instead, she gently says, 'Maybe we will go tomorrow Mama'. She then distracts Else by reading her the newspaper or showing her clips of Fred Astaire and Ginger Rogers videos on her laptop which Else very much enjoys. Grete does not fully understand what is going on in Else's brain but sees her agitation as some sort of longing for security and reassurance which is clearly felt more acutely at that time of day.

## Apraxia

In lay terms, apraxia is a malfunction of the brain which means that there is a disconnect between having the idea of doing something and actually doing it. Apraxia is a condition where the person finds it difficult to remember the correct order in which to do things. This affects their ability to perform a previously learned set of steps or movements, such as tying shoelaces or putting on clothes. Apraxia is common in Alzheimer's disease, usually appearing after impairments of memory and language are established. As someone's Alzheimer's progresses through the stages, their ability to perform certain activities of daily living such as bathing and getting dressed declines. In the middle/late stages of Alzheimer's disease, even activities such as walking and eating become more difficult. Due to the changes associated with apraxia, people living with Alzheimer's become at high risk of falling.

## Activity 2.4

### The five A's of Alzheimer's disease

Apraxia is one of five effects of Alzheimer's which are often referred to as the five A's. These are five common cognitive impairments seen in Alzheimer's disease as it progresses. They are amnesia (memory problems); aphasia (impaired communication); apraxia (loss of voluntary motor skills); agnosia (the loss of the ability to recognise objects faces, voices or places) and anomia (difficulty with finding the right words or names of everyday objects).

These are medical terms seldom used in everyday discourse. However, it is useful to be familiar with them because other professionals, the person or the person's carers might use them. The definitions and explanations provided here are minimal. Be sure to go to a reliable resource such as the NHS website and makes sure you understand what these terms mean in the context of people living with Alzheimer's disease and other forms of dementia. You will also see some websites refer to the '7 A's' of Alzheimer's. However, the five listed here are commonly used in respect of talking about dementia in the UK and it is, therefore, useful to know what they mean.

## Late/final stage

The final stage of Alzheimer's disease lasts, on average, one to three years but can be a much shorter period depending on other health issues. In the final stage of the disease dementia, symptoms are increasingly severe and incapacitating. During this stage, people become more vulnerable to infections, especially pneumonia, which is often the eventual cause of death. They are also at greater risk of pressure sores due to lack of mobility. Communicating pain through speech becomes difficult. The risk of depression increases. The risk of drug interactions from polypharmacy also increases. Memory and cognitive skills continue to worsen. Confusion and disorientation are more likely and significant personality changes are likely to take place including self-estrangement. Movement and motor skills generally are severely impaired. Therefore, standing, walking, swallowing and eating become difficult and will require assistance. Risk of dehydration increases during this stage. Bowel and bladder continence declines. As a consequence of these changes, people in the final stage of Alzheimer's usually require personal care both night and day. Despite the obvious deterioration in both physical and mental health, it is important that appropriate therapeutic interventions continue to be considered and that the tendency towards offering purely task-orientated and body-focused care is avoided.

The multiple, accumulative losses associated with the final stage of Alzheimer's epitomise what Laslett (1987) called the 'fourth age' – the period at the end of life characterised by 'dependency, decrepitude, and death'. Gilleard and Higgs (2010) have described the fourth age as 'ageing without agency', a bleak prospect that, unsurprisingly, most people dread as a way of spending the final period of their lives (Gilleard and Higgs, 2014, 2015). There is no avoiding the fact that the final stages of Alzheimer's can be a distressing period for the person and for those around them. It can be a harrowing experience to witness someone that you know go through this stage and it can evoke strong feelings of grief and anger, even repulsion or disgust. Whilst the person will require a high level of person-centred care and support, their family and those close to them will probably also need emotional, practical and spiritual support. However, everyone has their own way of coping, so if this is offered and turned down that should be accepted as their choice. They might change their minds later. The important thing is to make the offer.

## Vascular dementia

After Alzheimer's disease, vascular dementia is the second most common type of dementia in the UK. Vascular means relating to or affecting the blood vessels. Vascular dementia is usually caused by an acute, specific event such as a stroke or transient ischemic attack (TIA) in which blood flow to the brain has been interrupted. It also can develop more gradually over time from very small blockages or the slowing of blood flow. The most common form of vascular dementia is 'multi-infarct dementia'. 'Infarction' is the name for an (often small) stroke caused by a blockage in a blood vessel in the brain. This can also be called an ischemic stroke. 'Multi-infarct' basically means that the brain has been affected by multiple small strokes which have blocked the flow of blood to different parts of the brain. Vascular dementia can also be brought on by atrial fibrillation (irregular heart rhythms) and hypertension (high blood pressure). It is also linked to diabetes. The fact that African–Caribbean communities in the UK are at higher risk of vascular dementia is probably due to the greater prevalence of conditions such as diabetes and hypertension in those communities (Adelman, Blanchard and Livingston, 2009). By its nature, vascular dementia has more of a sudden onset. Its progression thereafter is usually step-like but accumulative (Cayton, Graham and Warner, 2002). As it progresses, it takes on more and more of the characteristics of Alzheimer's.

Unlike Alzheimer's disease, memory loss is not the typical first symptom of vascular dementia. Instead, people with vascular dementia can have different symptoms, depending on the area of the brain that is affected. The first symptoms to appear are often poor concentration, problems with communication, slowness of thought and difficulties with planning. There can be changes in mood which can sometimes be mistaken for depression. There can also be changes in behaviour and personality with the person sometimes becoming more aggressive. There can also be physical symptoms such as weakness or tremors.

The symptoms often continue to get worse and more impactful over time. Deterioration can sometimes be abrupt and sudden. How symptoms develop depends on the parts of the brain affected. Worsening of physical symptoms can include increasing difficulty with activities of daily living such as getting out of bed, personal care, walking and maintaining balance, with the risk of falls increasing. People can also experience a loss of bladder control (urinary incontinence). Vascular dementia can bring sleep disturbances. It is associated with obstructive sleep apnea. This is a serious sleep condition that can contribute to mood disorders and other cognitive complaints as well as excessive daytime sleepiness.

It is worth making the point that, with its links to cardiovascular health more generally, the risk of getting vascular dementia can be reduced (but not eliminated completely) by making certain lifestyle changes that promote heart health (BHF, 2018).

## Activity 2.5: Personal experiences

Alzheimer's Research UK have produced a short video 'Olive's story: living with vascular dementia'. Watch it for a more personal insight into how vascular dementia can affect somebody and those close to them. As she says, 'You don't know what you're going to lose next. You just have to wait and see.' www.youtube.com/watch?v=9luNs6AvQK8

Another account of vascular dementia – from a daughter's perspective – is provided by Chris Carling (2012). As we saw in Case Study 2.1, Chris's mum, Mary, was living with Alzheimer's disease. So it is interesting to see the comparison made. Chris writes:

Dad's diagnosis of 'vascular dementia' was just a label to start with. For all practical purposes he continued in the low, depressed state he had suffered for some while. Showing itself as 'not doing' – not saying much, not taking initiatives – vascular dementia can look like depression in the early stages. But Dad still seemed to inhabit the same world as me, he could tell fantasy from reality. As for Mum, though she did show some odd behaviour – with hindsight, quite a lot of odd behaviour, which became even odder with time – her spirit, determination and strong will meant that she could appear more normal than she almost certainly was. What is normal, after all?

Yes, each new incident made it clearer that something was definitely wrong, but in between were periods of apparent calm when Dad still joked and Mum seemed closer to her usual self. Or maybe our idea of her 'usual self' was shifting to accommodate her new behaviour.

Another factor may also have contributed: Mum and Dad were very good at putting on a convincing front. Good enough for us to take them at face value, accepting what they wanted to show us when we visited. We didn't know the full story of their day-to-day deterioration. Not until it was well advanced anyway (p. 186).

The two case studies illustrate how vascular dementia not only impacts on the person but also those close to them. Reflect upon the emotional and other adjustments that the person and those around them make when experiencing the effects of vascular dementia. What help or support do you think they need?

Unfortunately, there is currently no cure for vascular dementia nor a way to reverse the damage that has already happened. Medicines can be offered to treat the underlying cause of vascular dementia such as medication for high blood pressure or for high cholesterol which can help stop it from getting worse. Anti-depressant drugs can be prescribed where depression is also present. There are other non-medical interventions that can be used to manage the symptoms and promote better health and wellbeing. These will be covered in Chapter 6.

## Mixed dementia

Unfortunately, some people develop more than one type of dementia over their lifetime. This is referred to as 'mixed dementia' (Alzheimer's Society, 2021b). Specifically, the term 'mixed dementia' should only be applied to someone if they have clear clinical features of two types of disease that directly contribute to dementia symptoms. The most common mix is to have Alzheimer's and vascular dementia. However, there are other combinations of dementias that people live with. For example, to have Alzheimer's disease and dementia with Lewy bodies (DLB) (discussed in the following section) is not uncommon. The person will usually have one type that is predominant, but their symptoms will vary depending on the types of dementia that they have and which parts of their brain are most affected.

In the UK, at least one in every ten people with dementia is diagnosed as having more than one type. Although it needs pointing out that the fact that someone is living with more than one type of dementia is not always picked up and diagnosed accurately, so the actual incidence of mixed dementia could be higher (Dementia UK, n.d.a). Mixed dementia is much more common in older age groups such as those over 75 years old (Dementia Statistics, 2021b). Although it is often quite difficult to disentangle which type of dementia is causing which particular symptoms, identifying the underlying cause of dementia can help understand the pattern of progression of the condition and inform the choice of treatment. For example, people with Alzheimer's and vascular dementia can be given treatments to reduce the risk of further infarcts and potentially prevent ongoing brain damage from vascular causes. People with DLB are very sensitive to antipsychotic drugs. Therefore, even though such medication can have a calming effect on people living with Alzheimer's, in cases where someone has a combination of Alzheimer's disease and DLB this form of treatment should be avoided.

## Dementia with Lewy bodies

It is estimated that in the UK, 15% of people with dementia have DLB. DLB is the second commonest cause of degenerative dementia in older people after Alzheimer's disease and the third most common cause of dementia overall (Dementia Statistics, 2021b).

DLB is caused by abnormal protein structures called Lewy bodies (alpha-synuclein) that appear in nerve cells in the brain. The protein deposits in the brain obstruct chemical messages within the brain and disrupt the normal function. It is not yet known why Lewy bodies appear. DLB affects the brain's executive functions such as the ability to plan ahead and coordinate mental activities. It also impairs attention and alertness. Apart from causing loss of cognitive function DLB also has physiological features that resemble the symptoms of Parkinson's disease such as problems with walking and balance, rigid muscles, tremors, loss of facial expression and difficulties with speaking. People living with Lewy body dementia can also experience visual and auditory hallucinations. Half or more of people with Lewy body disease also develop signs and symptoms of Parkinson's disease. There is a strong overlap between the two conditions with the medical profession still researching the connections (Goldman et al., 2014; Jellinger, 2018). From the perspective of people with Parkinson's disease, it is estimated that about 50%–80% develop a type of dementia in the later stages and can have signs of Lewy bodies in their brains.

Unlike with Alzheimer's disease, where deficits in memory and concentration orientation are pretty constant from day to day, someone with DLB can be markedly different on different occasions. On some days, for example, a person with DLB will have a short episode of being very confused, which will then resolve. This pattern is typical of Lewy body dementia but is not common in Alzheimer's disease. These fluctuations can make the management and treatment of DLB quite difficult. The unpredictability and changeability of symptoms presents challenges for families and carers. It is more difficult to predict how the person is going to feel or behave on a day-to-day basis compared to someone with Alzheimer's disease.

## Activity 2.6

1    Check out a short video on the Rare Dementia Support YouTube Channel called 'Living with LBD: A short film' www.youtube.com/watch?v=Axn4FvlWFds
        This provides a brief but informative introduction to this particular form of dementia from the personal point of view of 'Roy'.
2    Go to the Dementia Alliance International website and check out the extract 'Peter Ashley: this is my life'. www.dementiaallianceinternational.org/peter-ashley-life/
        This extract provides a longer, more detailed personal written account by Peter Ashley of his learning about and dealing with discovering he had DLB. Peter's dementia activist approach is clear to see in this account.

As with all types of dementia, there is currently no cure for DLB. Symptoms can often be alleviated and managed by different medical and non-medical interventions. For some, Alzheimer's drugs can be helpful, whereas medication for Parkinson's can help people with DLB who display the motor symptoms such as tremor or rigidity. However, these drugs can increase confusion in others. As discussed earlier, people with DLB are very sensitive to some antipsychotic drugs. They can bring on side effects such as involuntary or uncontrollable movements, tremors and muscle contractions. Therefore, antipsychotic drugs should be avoided if at all possible. Non-medical interventions would include those offered to all people living with dementia (see Chapter 6). However, because of the Parkinsonian effects associated with DLB, physiotherapy and physical activity can be particularly helpful in maintaining mobility and helping the person (and their carers) to manage daily life. In the UK, the Lewy Body Society provides specialised advice and support for people living with the condition and their carers.

## Frontotemporal dementia

Frontotemporal dementia (FTD) is the name given to disorders that affect the frontal and temporal lobes of the brain. FTD is sometimes also known as Pick's disease. FTD is thought to be the second most common cause of dementia in the under 65s. It was originally given the name Pick's disease after the Czech neurologist and psychiatrist Arnold Pick who first identified the condition linking it to the frontal and temporal lobes of the brain. It is now mainly called FTD. As two-thirds of people with FTD are diagnosed with a subtype called 'behavioural variant frontotemporal dementia', often the abbreviation 'bvFTD' is used. The frontal and temporal lobes are at the front of the brain. They control important functions such as our behaviour and language. Damage in the frontal lobe part of the brain affects 'executive function' (the ability to control what the rest of the brain is doing). This includes planning, problem-solving, being able to make decisions, judgement, reasoning and organising.

Compared to Alzheimer's disease memory problems tend to show themselves later. The main problems that people living with FTD experience are either a change in their behaviour, a change in their personality or a change in their language. Behavioural symptoms include changes in motivation; the development of inappropriate (often disinhibited) social behaviour; showing behaviour that is more obsessive and compulsive; a loss of empathy; change in appetite, eating habits and diet and lack of insight. Symptoms get progressively worse and, in the later stages, the condition more closely resembles Alzheimer's disease.

## Case Study 2.3

Alzheimer's Research UK have put a short video called 'Urvashi's story: living with frontotemporal dementia' up on YouTube. The URL at the time of writing is www.youtube.com/watch?v=nPg6xyeloU0. At times, a difficult video to watch, it provides some key insights into what it is like to experience this disease. As the commentary to the video explains, 'Urvashi was almost relieved to learn that her husband's strange behaviour was not his fault, but caused by a disease. Frontotemporal dementia has turned their lives upside down.'

There are various other clips and videos available to watch online which portray different situations of people living with FTD. One to seek out, if possible, is a documentary made by the comedian and writer David Baddiel called 'The Trouble with Dad'. Baddiel's father Colin has been living with FTD for many years. The hour-long documentary, filmed over the course of a year, showed the reality of his father's life from the perspective of David Baddiel and other family members. It was broadcast on Channel Four TV in 2017. It shows the family having to adapt and manage the gradual deterioration in Colin's behaviour, which includes swearing, disinhibition and extreme rudeness. In an interview about the documentary, David Baddiel said 'if you can imagine Viz's Roger Mellie, a bit more sweary, and Welsh, that's my dad. And what the dementia has done is make that side of him – what you might call his anti-social side – grow like a malignant lesion, to the expense of all others.' Whilst Baddiel treats the topic with a lightness of touch and humour at times, there is no mistaking the difficulty of the challenges that living with FTD creates for Colin and those around him.

There is currently no cure for FTD and, in most cases, its progression cannot be slowed. However, whilst it is possible to manage some of the behavioural symptoms with medication, certain drugs (such as cholinesterase inhibitors) commonly used to treat other types of dementia are not recommended for people with FTD. The most effective way to manage symptoms is considered to be through behavioural and environmental interventions. A reassuring approach and distracting tactics are considered to be helpful in managing the behavioural and psychological problems associated with the disease. It is also useful to be able to identify and control known triggers to problematic behaviours.

## Alcohol-related dementia

In addition to many other health problems, the consumption of too much alcohol over a prolonged period of time can cause alcohol-related brain damage (ARBD). This can lead to the development of a form of dementia. Korsakoff's syndrome (also known as Wernicke–Korsakoff syndrome or just Korsakoff) is a chronic memory disorder caused by severe deficiency of thiamine (vitamin B1). Continued alcohol high levels of alcohol consumption will mean that the symptoms of dementia are likely to get progressively worse. However, if alcohol consumption stops completely, deterioration can be halted. It is often possible for some recovery to take place over time. Whilst Korsakoff's is considered a treatable condition, how successful the treatment is will depend on the degree of damage already done to the brain.

As well as memory Korsakoff's can affect other cognitive skills such as learning and reasoning, as well as personality, mood and social skills. As with other forms of dementia people with Korsakoff's can be prone to confabulation. The cognitive problems that people with Korsakoff's experience are often compounded by negative social reactions because of the connection with alcohol abuse. The combination of the stigma associated with dementia and the stigma associated with alcohol abuse effectively becomes a 'double stigma' and can lead to people with Korsakoff's experiencing discriminatory treatment. It is, perhaps, not difficult to see that if this particular form of dementia is considered to be self-induced and avoidable then it becomes easier to 'blame the victim'. However, such attitudes fail to take into account the complexities of ARBD. People with Korsakoff's vulnerability to double stigma needs to be recognised and challenged in order for them to receive the proper person-centred care, support and treatment that they need (Schölin et al., 2019).

## Rarer dementias

Most people living with dementia in the UK have Alzheimer's disease or vascular dementia. DLB, FTD and Korsakoff's are the next most common types but are rarer. However, there are many other rarer forms of dementia that social workers might encounter in their practice. These include posterior cortical atrophy, primary progressive aphasia and familial Alzheimer's disease (FAD), Creutzfeldt-Jakob Disease, Huntington's Disease and Normal Pressure Hydrocephalus. It is claimed that 30% of people living with the rarer forms of dementia initially receive an incorrect diagnosis (Rare Dementia Support Group, 2022). Because of their rarity, there tends to be both a widespread lack of understanding about these conditions and a shortage of specialised resources to support those affected. Because they all have their own patterns of progression, it is advisable to check the NHS website (www.nhs.uk/conditions/) for more specific information on causes, symptoms and treatments. For more information on support for people living with rarer forms of dementia see the Rare Dementia Support Group website (www.raredementiasupport.org).

## Comorbidities – not to be neglected

Diagnosing other health conditions – comorbidities – in people with dementia can be difficult and become more difficult as the severity of dementia increases especially as, amongst other things, communication becomes more difficult. However, another significant problem for people living with different forms of dementia is that their dementia diagnostic 'label'; be it 'Alzheimer's', 'Lewy bodies', 'Korsakoff's' or something else, can easily become their 'master status' (Doyle and Rubinstein, 2014). That is to say that, in health matters and in life generally, everything about them, their behaviour, their mood and so on becomes interpreted through the lens of their dementia, often to the exclusion of all else. The diagnosis of dementia defines who they are. For example, if the person is groaning or shouting, it is attributed to their dementia, if they appear agitated or listless it is attributed to their dementia, if they lose their appetite or fall, it is attributed to their dementia and so on and so forth. In such circumstances, the effect of dementia being someone's master status means that signs and symptoms of other health conditions can be misdiagnosed or overlooked altogether.

The fact is that many people living with dementia are likely to have multiple health conditions and impairments and therefore more likely to have complex health needs, particularly as they get older and the disease progresses. Almost seven in ten people living with dementia have one or more other health conditions (Public Health England, 2019a). 44% of people living with dementia have a diagnosis of hypertension; between 17% and 20% have a diagnosis of diabetes, stroke or TIA, coronary heart disease (CHD) or depression. Between 9% and 11% have a diagnosis of Parkinsonism, chronic obstructive pulmonary disease (COPD) or asthma (Public Health England, 2019a). It is estimated that the incidence of depression is at last 30% in people with vascular dementia and with Alzheimer's disease, and over 40% in dementia associated with Parkinson's disease (Kitching, 2015). Older adults (85 and over) with dementia and medium or high dependency needs are more likely to have at least two other comorbidities. The proportion of those who are 85 and over and who have dementia and at least two other health conditions is projected to increase from 58.8% in 2015 to 81.2% in 2035 (Kingston, Comas-Herrera and Jagger, 2018). The most common comorbidities which lead to hospital admission in the UK are preventable conditions such as falls, fractured hips as well as urinary and chest infections (Dementia Statistics, 2021a; Scrutton and Barancati, 2016).

It should be recognised that people living with dementia are, in general, more likely to develop comorbidities than people who do not have dementia. Therefore, it is important that 'dementia' does not become their health master status with health and care professionals failing to properly investigate and diagnose other health problems as a consequence. The diagnosis and timely treatment of other health conditions will help the person with the experience of living with dementia. However, the presence of chronic comorbidities alongside dementia means that the health and care support needed by the person with dementia will be complex and will require regular reviews by the person's GP and any other health and social care professional involved.

## Summary of key points

- There are over 100 types of dementia.
- In order to work effectively as part of a multi-disciplinary team, social workers need to know the difference between the different types of dementia and to be conversant with the relevant medical terminology.
- People often find it useful to have a specific medical diagnosis and to understand what that means in terms of the progression and treatment of the disease.
- In the UK, Alzheimer's disease accounts for between 60% and 70% of all dementias. The longer someone lives the greater the chance of getting the disease.
- Roughly 5% of people with Alzheimer's in the UK are under 65.
- People with Down's syndrome have a higher risk of developing Alzheimer's disease.
- Vascular dementia is the second most common type of dementia in the UK.
- The risk of getting vascular dementia can be reduced by making lifestyle changes that promote heart health.
- In the UK, at least one in every ten people with dementia is diagnosed as having more than one type of dementia. Mixed dementia is much more common in older age groups, such as those over 75 years old.

- With more people living longer and with more people developing different forms of dementia, management of polypharmacy is a growing issue.
- Around 15% of people with dementia in the UK have DLB which is the second most common cause of degenerative dementia in older people after Alzheimer's disease and the third most common cause of dementia overall.
- FTD is estimated to be the second most common cause of dementia in the under 65s.
- Korsakoff's syndrome is a form of dementia associated with alcohol abuse. If diagnosed early and treated properly it can be reversible.
- Nearly 70% of people living with dementia have one or more other health conditions such as hypertension, diabetes, CHD, stroke and depression. These comorbidities are not always picked up, often because the diagnosis of dementia has become the person's master status.

## Further reading

The best and most accessible sources of up to date information on different types of dementia are:

The Alzheimer's Society website: www.alzheimers.org.uk/about-dementia/types-dementia

The NHS Website: www.nhs.uk/conditions/dementia/about/?tabname=about-dementia

UCL Dementia Research Centre: www.ucl.ac.uk/drc/

The Rare Dementia Support Group www.raredementiasupport.org and the Lewy Body Society www.lewybody.org/ are organisations whose websites are useful to learn more about the less common forms of dementia and about what support is available for people living with these conditions.

*The Dementia Guide: Living Well after Diagnosis* published by the Alzheimer's Society (2017) in paperback form and online provides a free and very accessible overview of all aspects of living with dementia, including sections on different types, treatments and services available at www.alzheimers.org.uk/publications-about-dementia/the-dementia-guide

# 3

# DEMENTIA IN CONTEXT

By the end of this chapter, you should have an understanding of:

- The demographic, public health and economic contexts in which social work practice with dementia takes place.
- The legislative and policy context in which social work practice with people living with dementia takes place in the UK.

## Introduction

In Chapter 1, it was highlighted how an overconcentration on the number of people with dementia and on the costs of supporting them risks creating an 'other-ing' effect. Too much emphasis on the statistics of dementia, and the actual people living with it can easily be become regarded as a growing, faceless and burdensome mass who threaten to overwhelm our health, social and economic systems. Reference was made to the 'burden', 'zombie' and 'war on dementia' discourses in this respect. Nevertheless, in order to understand both the scale and nature of the challenges facing health and social care systems around the world, it is necessary to have a certain amount of quantitative information about dementia in order to put the challenges it raises into context. However, in this chapter, the facts and figures are provided with the caveat that it always needs to be remembered that behind each of the statistics lies an individual's personal, lived experience.

## The demographic and public health context

Two major demographic trends both in the UK and globally are that societies are becoming, on average, progressively older and they are increasingly more diverse in terms of ethnicity. Both of these trends have a bearing on the prevalence and

DOI: 10.4324/9781003191667-4

incidence of dementia globally and, more specifically, in the UK. Ageing is of particular importance because the longer that we live the greater are our chances of developing a form of dementia (Stephan and Brayne, 2014). More recently established ethnic communities in countries like the UK and USA are, on average, younger. However, these communities are settling, expanding and beginning to age at a faster rate than the predominantly white host populations. This means that countries like the UK and USA will see more and more people living with dementia from different ethnic backgrounds. This throws up its own challenges in terms of raising awareness and enabling access to suitable services (Boise, 2014).

## The global picture

In global terms, it is estimated that, currently, around 50 million people have some form of dementia, with nearly 10 million new 'cases' being diagnosed every year. The overall number of people living with dementia globally is projected to reach 82 million people in 2030 and 152 million people by 2050. As explained earlier, a major contributory factor in this rise is that more and more people are living longer. This trend is linked to standards of living rising and medical care improving around the world. Currently, it is estimated that between 5% and 8% of the world's population aged over 60 is living with some type of dementia. Globally, Alzheimer's disease is the most common form of dementia making up around 60%–70% of all cases (WHO, 2020). The economic impact in terms of direct medical and social care costs and the indirect costs associated with informal care is significant. This is put into context somewhat dramatically on the Social Care Institute for Excellence website which states:

> According to Alzheimer's Disease International, the total estimated worldwide cost of dementia was US $1 trillion in 2018. If dementia care were a country, it would be the world's 18th largest economy. If dementia care were a company, it would be the world's largest by annual revenue exceeding Apple, Google and Exxon.
>
> *(SCIE, 2020)*

In 2015, the total global societal cost of dementia was estimated to be 1.1% of the global gross domestic product (SCIE, 2020). When put in these terms, it is impossible to avoid talking about the growing numbers of people living with dementia without taking into account the costs of caring for and supporting them. The steadily growing number of people with dementia is a major public health issue that requires a significant public funding response. In this context, it is not difficult to see why a major consideration of dementia strategies around the world is to lower the risks of developing dementia wherever possible (World Health Organisation, 2017). Delaying the onset of dementia for as many people as possible and reducing the overall prevalence of dementia in the population will help release more resources for those actually living with dementia who need to use health and social care services (Stephan and Brayne, 2014).

## Numbers of people with dementia in the UK

According to Age UK (n.d.), only 43% of people living with a form of dementia have actually been diagnosed as having it, so statistics cannot be too precise. However, it is estimated that in 2021, more than 920,000 people in the UK were living with dementia. The vast majority (over 880,000 people) were aged 65 and over. Although an estimated 40,000 people under the age of 65 are also living with a form of dementia, most commonly young-onset Alzheimer's disease. There are over 200,000 new cases of dementia diagnosed in the UK each year (SCIE, 2020). One in six people over the age of 80 have dementia and NHS England (2021) estimates that one in three people will care for a person with dementia in their lifetime. As explained, the main driver behind the increases in the number of people developing dementia is that, on average, people are living longer. Deaths due to different types of dementia (notably Alzheimer's disease) are now the main cause of death in England and Wales, accounting for nearly 13% of all deaths registered (NHS, n.d.).

## Diversity

Roughly two-thirds of people living with dementia in the UK (over 600,000) are women.

Alzheimer's disease and other dementias are now the leading cause of death in women in the UK. In 2018, 16.5% of women died due to some form of dementia. For men, it was 8.7%. One of the main reasons for the greater prevalence of dementia (and mortality rate) among women is their longer life expectancy compared to men (Dementia Statistics, 2021c). Dementia also has a greater impact on women as carers for people living with dementia. The majority of people (60%–70%) providing informal care for people with dementia are women. This amounts to roughly 700,000 unpaid carers (SCIE, 2020). Women are also more than twice as likely to provide care for someone for over 5 years and 24 hours a day (Dementia Statistics, 2021c). Therefore, not only do more women than men end up as carers, they perform this role, on average, for longer and more intensively. The fact that there are more women living with dementia than men and also that they are more likely to be caring for others with dementia than men has led to them being described as a 'marginalised majority' (Alzheimer's Research UK, 2015), because the double impact of dementia on women's lives, especially as they grow older, has yet to be fully acknowledged.

It is estimated that there are over 25,000 people from black and minority ethnic (BAME) groups in England and Wales living with dementia. This figure is predicted to rise to nearly 50,000 by 2026 and to over 172,000 people by 2051 (SCIE, 2020). The proportion of people from BAME communities who are affected by dementia will increase more rapidly than in the white population. Whilst it is estimated that the number of people with dementia across the whole UK population will double over the next 40 years, the number of people affected by dementia from BAME communities will increase nearly sevenfold. According to Cheston and Bradbury (2018: 1):

> By 2051, there will be six times as many Black Caribbean cases, 12 times as many Indian cases, 22 times as many Bangladeshi cases and 45 times as many Black African cases of dementia compared to 2001. This differential increase in the numbers of people affected by dementia is largely due to two factors: – Dementia is more common amongst Asian and Black Caribbean communities, at least in part because high blood pressure, diabetes, stroke and heart disease, which are risk factors for dementia, are more common. In addition, social factors, such as fewer years spent in education, lower levels of income and lower socio-economic status (all of which have been associated with dementia risk) may accentuate the risks for some BAME communities. – People who settled in the UK as young adults in the 1960s, 70s and 80s are only now reaching an age where there is a significantly higher risk of dementia.

An important point to make about the first factor mentioned by Chester and Bradbury is that due to cultural factors such as the stigma attached to mental illness, the incidence of dementia in certain BAME communities might well be significantly under presented and therefore underdiagnosed compared to that in the white population of the UK (All-Party Parliamentary Group on Dementia, 2013; Khan, 2015). In terms of the final point they make, there are more recent groups of immigrants to the UK than those mentioned, for example, from Southern and Eastern Europe, Central and South America. People from these groups will also start to show a greater incidence of dementia as those populations age. Not only are BAME communities growing as a proportion of the UK population they are also becoming more diverse (Khan, 2015). Therefore, with the prevalence of dementia increasing at a much higher rate within all BAME communities, it is recognised that campaigns need to be specifically targeted at these communities in order to raise awareness about dementia, challenge stigma, provide information about the availability of services and to tackle modifiable risk factors where possible (All-Party Parliamentary Group on Dementia, 2013).

## Cost

In 2019, it was estimated that the total cost to the UK economy of supporting people with dementia was £34.7 billion, which was more than the combined costs of looking after people with cancer and heart disease. Health care for people with dementia accounted for 14% of the total costs in the UK (£4.9 billion), whereas social care (publicly and privately funded) and unpaid care accounted for 45% (£15.7 billion) and 40% (£13.9 billion), respectively, of the total costs.

The total cost of dementia care in the UK is projected to grow from £34.7 billion in 2019 to £94.1 billion in 2040 – an increase of 172%. The percentage spent on social care out of the total costs of dementia care will rise slightly from 45% in

2019 to 48% in 2040 (Wittenberg et al., 2019). It is argued that in respect of the amount spent on social care, people living with dementia fare badly in comparison with those with other illnesses like cancer or heart disease, more of whose care is funded free at the point of delivery by the NHS. A diagnosis of dementia does not necessarily mean someone will qualify for NHS continuing healthcare (CHC) or NHS-funded nursing care (FNC) (see Chapter 6). Because much care for dementia is designated 'social care' this means that, apart from in Scotland, access to local authority-funded social care requires a means-test. As a consequence, many people pay for all their care privately.

In 2014, 61.3% of people with dementia over 65 in the UK were living in the community (a total of 493,639). When people with dementia remain in the community, it is found that their social care costs can rise sharply as the disease gets worse. In 2014, the annual average cost of care was around £3,100 for mild dementia, £7,800 for moderate dementia and £10,300 for severe dementia (Prince et al., 2014). As the severity of dementia increases, so does the likelihood of living in a care home. In the future, a higher proportion of people with dementia will live in care homes than will be supported in the community (Prince et al., 2014). In 2014, 311,730 people with dementia were living in either residential care or nursing homes (38.7%). The cost of living in a care home varies both across the four nations of the UK and within the four nations. How much someone pays depends on where they live, the type of care needed, their assets such as savings and property and the charges of the particular care home provider. At the time of writing, the majority of people with dementia currently have to self-fund until their assets fall below the threshold of £23,250. In 2021, the average monthly cost of living in a residential care home was £2,816, whilst living in a care home with nursing care costs on average £3,552 p.m. (carehome.co.uk, 2021). Taking all those with dementia receiving care together, they will, on average, pay £100,000 over their lifetime for care (Alzheimer's Society, 2021c).

In general terms, a diagnosis of dementia generally means a steadily rising financial cost to the individual, to any relatives who agree to top up care home fees (third-part top ups) and to the local authority and NHS.

## The state of health and social care in England

The Care Quality Commission (CQC), which regulates and inspects health and social care services in England, produces an annual report on the state of health care and adult social care in England. At the time of writing, its most recent report covered the years 2019–20 (CQC, 2020a). This was a period where health and social care was significantly impacted by the Government having to respond to the COVID-19 pandemic. Health and social care services were stretched more than usual for all service users. However, certain observations did not make for very good reading for those with dementia and who need care.

First, the report highlighted that there were generally difficulties across the country for people who needed residential care with nursing. CQC flagged as a related issue the lack of suitable provision for people with high support needs, including people living with dementia. Second, in 2019, CQC conducted an adult inpatient survey, which asked more than 75,000 people about their experiences at acute NHS trusts. The findings revealed that people with dementia were one of the groups who reported poorer experiences of care than others. The impact of the pandemic showed itself in several ways. CQC highlighted that the system of remote care (for example, assessments via Zoom) did not work particularly well for many living with dementia. GPs were reluctant to visit care homes and nearly a third of care home leaders found it difficult to access GP services on behalf of the people they care for which obviously included older people and those with dementia. The CQC concluded that, as a consequence, those in residential adult social care settings might have been at greater risk from general health problems being left untreated, as well as from COVID-19.

When CQC conducted a survey into the experiences of hospital inpatients in 2020, the responses to several of the questions, indicated that people living with different forms of dementia had worse experiences:

> They were least likely to say they were involved in decisions about their care or received answers to questions that they could 'always' understand. They were least likely to 'always' understand staff who were wearing PPE. Among groups with long-term health conditions, they had by far the lowest rate of feeling able to keep in touch with their families during their stay in hospital. 23% said they 'never' spoke with friends or family while in hospital.
>
> *(CQC, 2020a: 49)*

To combat the isolation caused by lockdown measures, some care home providers provided people with equipment such as computer tablets or smartphones in order to enable them to communicate with relatives and friends. CQC observed that 'some residents needed significant support to use digital platforms – and some people with dementia were unable to share the benefits' (CQC, 2020a: 78). So, overall, in what was a sector under stress with many people's needs unmet or not met fully, it appears that people living with dementia were often the group who fared worse. However, there were examples of good practice highlighted, including those provided in Case Study 3.1.

## Case Study 3.1:   Maintaining safe social contact during lockdown

> We spoke to Sarah, whose mother, Lesley, has Alzheimer's disease and lives in a specialist dementia unit at a care home. Lesley is cared for by specialist nurses and care assistants, as well as support from a dementia consultant several times a year and her GP when needed. Sarah and other family members used to visit

Lesley frequently, and they feel that Lesley is happy in her home and receives good care from the friendly and helpful staff.

Earlier this year, the home where Lesley lives had some cases of COVID-19 and decided to go into lockdown before the official government advice came out. Sarah was supportive of this, although it meant she was no longer able to visit her mother because she understood the actions were being taken to keep people safe.

Sarah and her family called the home every day to check how Lesley was doing, and the staff were always happy to provide an update and support Lesley to speak to her family directly over the phone. When it became clear that lockdown was going to last for a longer period, the care home arranged for video calling between the family and Lesley, and supported Lesley to use this. The staff noticed that Lesley would offer her family tea and cake over the video call, and suggested to Sarah that they arrange to call at teatime, so they could all have tea and cake together. They arranged a special tea at Easter and decorated an Easter bonnet for Lesley to wear.

When lockdown measures started to ease, the care home arranged for garden visits so that Sarah and other family members could see Lesley in person. The staff made sure that safety measures were in place, such as providing gloves and masks, allowing one visitor at a time, and keeping to physical distancing advice.

During lockdown, Lesley's consultant from the hospital was able to carry out her quarterly assessment by video-link and later commented that he was impressed with how well the staff knew Lesley's condition and the level of detail they were able to provide.

Sarah told us that she 'could not fault the care that [Lesley] had been given by the staff pre and during COVID'. She is fully confident and it helps to know that her mother is being so well cared for in these difficult times (CQC, 2020a: 36).

Key factors in maintaining safe social contact during lockdown appeared to be the efforts by the staff to maintain channels of communication with both relatives and other professionals; being innovative and trying to balance the need for safety with a need to attend to Lesley's social and emotional needs. Many people with dementia living in care homes were having to cope with their disease and with isolation often unable to understand what was causing it.

Before the lockdowns of 2020 and 2021 created their own problems, there were other issues that needed addressing in respect of people living with dementia in care homes. For example, the number of people from BAME communities living with dementia is rising rapidly and, as a consequence, the number of people from these communities moving into care homes is also increasing sharply. However, according to Milne and Smith (2015), due to factors such as lack of training and cultural competence amongst the staff, older people with dementia from BAME communities in care homes are one of 'the most marginalised and invisible groups' of service users in the UK (p. 212). This, Milne and Smith explain, is because people from these groups:

> . . . experience multiple disadvantages arising from having a stigmatised condition, living in a setting that may not meet their needs effectively, and that is away from their family, community and social cultural norms (p. 212).

Apart from ensuring better training to provide culturally appropriate care, Milne and Smith argue that policymakers and care professionals need a more accurate picture of the actual numbers and characteristics of different BAME groups living with dementia in care homes. The issue of care homes highlights more general questions about how the social system responds to the increasing numbers of people from BAME groups with dementia. Given the demographic, social and health trends discussed earlier, it is an issue with several dimensions to it but one of growing importance for policymakers and practitioners.

The CQC report also highlighted some more general but fundamental problems with the system of adult social care in the UK which have been ongoing for decades. As the King's Fund (2021) put it:

> The social care system is not fit for purpose and is failing the people who rely on it, with high levels of unmet need and providers struggling to deliver the quality of care that older and disabled people have a right to expect. These combine to place great pressures on families and carers. (www.kingsfund.org.uk/projects/positions/adult-social-care-funding-and-eligibility)

The necessary reform of the adult social care system has been avoided and put back by successive governments in the UK. In England, many reports have been published over the years but very little has been done, leaving problems with both the quantity and quality of service provision as well as unresolved issues in respect of funding and affordability (NAO, 2021). Therefore, social work with people living with dementia currently takes place in a context where the social care system is not funded adequately nor organised well enough to meet all the needs of the ever-growing numbers of people living with dementia and those who care for them in a fair and equitable manner.

## Summary of key points

- In the UK and globally societies are becoming, on average, progressively older and they are becoming increasingly more diverse in terms of ethnicity.
- The longer we live, the greater our chances of developing dementia, which is creating a major public health issue worldwide.
- The overall number of people living with dementia globally is projected to reach 82 million people in 2030 and 152 million people by 2050.
- It is estimated that in 2021 more than 920,000 people in the UK were living with dementia. The vast majority were aged 65 and over, with an estimated 40,000 people under the age of 65 are also living with a form of dementia. There are over 200,000 new cases of dementia diagnosed in the UK each year.
- Roughly two-thirds of people living with dementia in the UK are women.
- Over the next 40 years, the number of people affected by dementia from BAME communities in the UK will increase nearly sevenfold.
- The total cost of dementia care in the UK is projected to grow from £34.7 billion in 2019 to £94.1 billion in 2040.
- In 2014, 61.3% of people with dementia over 65 in the UK were living in the community and 38.7% in some form of care home.
- In the UK, people living with dementia requiring social care will, on average, pay £100,000 over their lifetime for that care.
- Currently, people with dementia are not served that well by the adult social care system compared to other groups. People with dementia from BAME communities in care homes are further marginalised within the system.

## Global responses

The rising number of people around the world who are living with dementia are now recognised as a significant public health issue internationally. At the global level, the response has been led and coordinated by the WHO. In 2012, the WHO (in conjunction with Alzheimer's Disease International) published *Dementia: A Public Health Priority*, in which they declared that:

Dementia is overwhelming not only for the people who have it, but also for their caregivers and families. It is one of the major causes of disability and dependency among older people worldwide. There is lack of awareness and understanding of dementia, at some level, in most countries, resulting in stigmatization, barriers to diagnosis and care, and impacting caregivers, families and societies physically, psychologically and economically. Dementia can no longer be neglected but should be considered a part of the public health agenda in all countries.

*(WHO, 2012: 2)*

The WHO was making dementia a public health priority and was calling for concerted action, not just on a national but an international scale. It urged member states to include dementia on their public health agendas. Key messages that WHO wanted to disseminate were that:

Key messages

- People live for many years after the onset of symptoms of dementia. With appropriate support, many can and should be enabled to continue to engage and contribute within society and have a good quality of life.
- Dementia is overwhelming for the caregivers and adequate support is required for them from the health, social, financial and legal systems.
- Countries must include dementia on their public health agendas. Sustained action and coordination is required across multiple levels and with all stakeholders – at international, national, regional and local levels.
- People with dementia and their caregivers often have unique insights to their condition and life. They should be involved in formulating the policies, plans, laws and services that relate to them.
- The time to act is now by:

  - promoting a dementia-friendly society globally;
  - making dementia a national public health and social care priority worldwide;
  - improving public and professional attitudes to, and understanding of, dementia;
  - investing in health and social systems to improve care and services for people with dementia and their caregivers;
  - increasing the priority given to dementia in the public health research agenda (WHO, 2012: 4).

These elements of the WHO plan of action are now embedded in many national dementia strategies, including those of the four UK countries. In 2013, the UK hosted a G8 Dementia Summit which ended with a signed declaration of shared commitment from all the participating stakeholders and countries (G8 UK, 2013). These included calls to:

- . . . the WHO and OECD (Organisation for Economic Co-operation and Development) to identify dementia as an increasing threat to global health and support countries to strengthen health and social care systems to improve care and services for people with dementia;

- . . . the UN Independent Expert on the enjoyment of all human rights by older persons to integrate the perspective of older people affected by dementia into their work;
- . . . all sectors to treat people affected by dementia with dignity and respect, and to enhance their contribution to dementia prevention, care and treatment where they can; and
- . . . civil society to continue and to enhance global efforts to reduce stigma, exclusion and fear.

Of particular relevance to social work, we can see that the signatories were calling for responses to dementia that improved health and social care services, promoted human rights, reduced stigma and social exclusion and wanted people affected by dementia not only treated with dignity and respect but to be involved in shaping policy and practice. The point about reducing stigma and fear harks back to the discussion in Chapter 1 about the need to change traditional narratives about dementia. However, the complexities of meeting this challenge are evident from statements from the WHO and other bodies which, for example, talk in terms of dementia as 'overwhelming' caregivers and 'dementia as an increasing threat to global health'. One particular challenge is how to stress the urgency of responding to dementia without couching calls to do so in language that risks stigmatising those living with it.

In March 2015, WHO organised the first Ministerial Conference on the Global Action against Dementia with participants from 89 Member States. The conference concluded with a 'Call to Action' that was endorsed by participants. Its key themes were: accelerating focus on dementia risk reduction; strategic approaches for dementia research; living well with dementia; improving dementia awareness and reducing stigma; strengthening global leadership and a call for action, which mainly reiterated the action points made in the earlier report World Health Organization (2015a). In the same year, the WHO called for member states to put in place a human rights-based approach for people living with dementia. This was to incorporate the principles set out in the 'PANEL' framework: Participation; Accountability; Non-discrimination; Empowerment and Legality (WHO, 2015b).

Following the 70th World Health Assembly in 2017, the WHO launched more global dementia initiatives. These include:

## Global Dementia Observatory

The WHO Global Dementia Observatory is an interactive web-based data and knowledge exchange platform. It collates and disseminates data from countries on key dementia indicators in order to facilitate countries to strengthen their systems to support people with dementia and their carers.

## *iSupport*

iSupport is an online support programme for carers of people with dementia. It is designed to support dementia carers to provide better care, with less detrimental consequences for their own health, whilst helping them to take better care of the person with dementia. WHO put a video on YouTube www.youtube.com/watch?v=_g2KMgjukzs explaining how it works.

## *Global Action Plan*

Delegates at the 70th World Health Assembly in Geneva, Switzerland, voted to adopt a Global Action Plan on the public health response to dementia (World Health Organisation, 2017). Its overall goal is to 'improve the lives of people with dementia, their carers and families, while decreasing the impact of dementia on them as well as on communities and countries'. The WHO Plan has seven areas for action: dementia as a public health priority; dementia awareness and friendliness; risk reduction; diagnosis, treatment, care, and support; support for carers; information systems and research and innovation. The Plan also includes seven cross-cutting principles to improve the lives of those living with dementia and their carers and to reduce the impact of dementia on society. These principles are about promoting:

1   Human rights of people with dementia.
2   Empowerment and engagement of people living with dementia and their carers.
3   Evidence-based dementia risk reduction and care.
4   Multi-sectoral collaboration on the public health response to dementia.
5   Universal health and social care coverage for dementia.
6   Equity, with special reference made to gender sensitivity.
7   Appropriate attention to dementia prevention, cure and care.

The Global Action Plan on Dementia has been praised for being comprehensive and also reflecting a high level of collective effort and solidarity amongst dementia advocates and organisations. However, doubts have been expressed about whether some countries, especially lower- and middle-income countries (LMICs), have the leadership and resources to deliver on all aspects of the agenda.

With any awareness-raising campaigns, some notes of caution need to be sounded. As was highlighted in Chapter 1, public health campaigns that set out to destigmatise dementia can sometimes inadvertently contribute to the 'benevolent othering' of the very groups of people they want to destigmatise. So this aspect needs to be handled carefully. However, the worst-case scenario, as Cahill (2020) explains:

> is that awareness campaigns and risk reduction programmes will yield no dividends, prevalence rates especially in LMICs will continue to soar, the public health approach will generate a culture of blame and shame thereby

reinforcing stigma and many countries will produce glossy policy plans but fail abysmally in terms of their implementation and evaluation.

*(p. 199)*

This section has highlighted the considerable burst of activity from world bodies over the past decade that have recognised that dementia must be made a public health priority internationally. The vision and action plan for responding to the challenges of dementia globally have been rightly praised. However, ensuring that national dementia strategies effectively put the WHO principles and actions points into practice on the ground is an ongoing challenge.

## National policy responses to dementia

In the UK, oversight of social care and aspects of healthcare is devolved to each of the four nations. England, Wales, Scotland and Northern Ireland have formulated their own national dementia strategies which are significantly informed by the principles, values and action points contained in the various WHO reports and calls for action. As a consequence, they have much in common.

## Activity 3.1

Depending on where you live locate and read your own country's dementia strategy.

- The Welsh Government published the *Dementia Action Plan for Wales 2018–2022* in 2018.
- The Scottish Government published *Scotland's National Dementia Strategy 2017–2020* in June 2017.
- In England, the Department of Health published *the Prime Minister's challenge on dementia 2020* in 2015.
- The Department of Health in Northern Ireland published *Improving dementia services in Northern Ireland – a regional strategy* in 2011. At the time of writing, this is yet to be updated. However, the Northern Ireland Executive ran the Dementia Services Programme, 'Dementia Together NI' from 2013 to 2017.

Make sure that you locate the most up-to-date plan for your country. It might have been revised or updated since the time of writing this book. Identify where you think social work has a part to play in enacting the strategy.

## *The evolution of policy on dementia*

Historically, provision for older people with mental illness in the UK has been given low priority by successive governments and, as a consequence, standards and availability of specialist provision have not been particularly good. In England, as recently as 2002, reports by the Audit Commission (2000, 2002) had flagged up that practice and provision were inconsistent across the country and, in some areas, inadequate. It was found that GPs and primary care staff were not given sufficient support and that specialist help and training were often limited. Many areas lacked specialist teams and there was a lack of good quality information about dementia and dementia services. Apart from problems getting the right advice and information, carers reported having difficulties accessing respite care.

However, for the reasons explained earlier in this chapter, it was clear that there was a pressing need to respond to the issues associated with growing numbers of people living with dementia. Consequently, in 2009, the Labour government published the country's first strategy aimed at dementia – *The National Dementia Strategy: Living Well with Dementia* (Department of Health, 2009). The three broad aims of the strategy were to ensure better knowledge about dementia and remove the stigma that surrounds it; to ensure that people with dementia are properly diagnosed and to develop a range of services for people with dementia and their carers that fully meets their changing needs over time. This was broken down into 17 more specific objectives. However, in 2010, a new Coalition government came into power replacing Labour. In *Quality outcomes for people with dementia: building on the work of the National Dementia Strategy* (Department of Health, 2010a), the Coalition government stated their intention to build on the previous year's strategy, but said that they wanted to focus on the following priorities:

- good-quality early diagnosis and intervention for all;
- improved quality of care in general hospitals;
- living well with dementia in care homes and
- reduced use of antipsychotic medication.

This publication served as a reminder that the drive to promote 'quality outcomes for people with dementia' was part of a more general health and social care agenda by the Coalition government which was 'about improving outcomes; ensuring autonomy, accountability, democratic legitimacy and improving efficiency' (p. 5). The point about improving efficiency is worth noting because the Coalition government came into power in the wake of the financial crisis of 2007–8. A major part of their programme was about reducing public spending. At the same time, the government (and, in particular, the then Prime Minister David Cameron) was promoting the idea of the 'Big Society'. Based around the concept of encouraging greater personal and family responsibility, voluntarism and community activism, when in the context of government austerity, the Big Society was, for many, regarded as trying to get vital public services 'on the cheap' (BBC, 2010). England's first *National Dementia Strategy* was therefore launched in a general climate of public spending cuts, for some, this was not conducive to achieving the desired outcomes (Ogden, 2017).

## Dementia and personalisation

From the 2000s onwards, successive governments in the UK have promoted an agenda of personalisation in adult social care, based on the idea of promoting choice through the use of direct payments and individual budgets (Carr, 2010).

Social workers were positioned as key professionals in making this happen for users of adult care services (SCIE, 2010).

In a report by the King's Fund (2006), it was reported that many informal carers believed that their workload and stress levels were already too high to cope without taking on direct payments. It was felt that, realistically, people living with dementia and their carers needed specialist support if they were to take the direct payments option. In 2011, the Alzheimer's Society (UK) produced a report on the use of personal budgets for people with dementia and their carers (Lakey and Saunders, 2014). Whilst it confirmed that personal budgets could offer benefits, it stated that they were not suitable for everyone, at least not without some adaptation, preferably made with the involvement of people with dementia and their carers. It was felt that other options needed to be made available, that the market should be better developed to deliver a range of different types of dementia services and that people with dementia and their carers needed to be provided with timely and appropriate information for the system to work for them properly. In the same year, the Department of Health (2011a) flagged up where progress was being made in this respect. However, at that time, it was evident that there was still much to be done to increase the take up of direct payments and for the system to make personalised care and support a reality for people with dementia (Department of Health, 2011a).

### The 'Prime Minister's challenge on dementia'

In 2012, the 'Prime Minister's challenge on dementia' (DH, 2012) was published. It provided a progress check on the *National Dementia Strategy* that had been launched three years previously and set a challenge to deliver major improvements in dementia care and research by 2015. Three champion groups were set up to focus on the main areas for action: driving improvements in health and care, creating dementia-friendly communities and improving dementia research. Case Study 3.2 provides an illustration of one of those areas.

## Case Study 3.2: A dementia-friendly city – York

The Prime Minister's challenge used a project in York to create a 'dementia-friendly city' as a case study (DH, 2012: 14). The project was carried out and reported on by the Joseph Rowntree Foundation (JRF, 2012). An extract is provided here.

## People

'I would like support from the people around me – my GP, vicar, my family – but they don't know what to do or say.'

People with dementia rely on others, to varying degrees, throughout their dementia lives. The critical people are partners, families, carers, neighbours, everyday service providers (such as shopkeepers, the milkman), as well as health and social care workers (and particularly GPs). What the people around them know about dementia, their attitudes to it, what they say and how they act, are critical to making people feel confident or otherwise. Carers are crucial for many people with dementia, and most care is provided within the family by a spouse or children or other close family members. It is important to provide support for carers to enable them to care, but also to recognise that they sometimes have a different view of the world from the person for whom they are caring.

The role of GPs is central to supporting people with dementia through early diagnosis and advice, not just about the long-term prognosis and care options, but also about staying well and engaged through the earlier stages. GPs' new lead in clinical commissioning through the NHS reforms means that their understanding and knowledge of dementia is even more important for the future. As a result of attending the project's sounding board event, the Vale of York Clinical Commissioning Group's lead GP on mental health and dementia recognised the value of training receptionists in her practice. This shows the immediate impact key people can have in creating dementia-friendly communities.

A sample of the key project findings about people:

- Increasing awareness of dementia and changing our attitude towards it can help to remove the stigma many people feel. This may help people to talk about their experience, to engage more in society and to ask for the help they need.
- Supporting carers and the families of people with dementia is essential to supporting people themselves.
- A consistent approach and response to diagnosis by GPs, and better sign-posting would increase confidence and support people in the community for longer (p. 4).

## Comment

The case study is reproduced here in order to underline the point that, whilst health and social care services are important, whole communities need to become 'dementia friendly' if people living with dementia are to live as lives that are as full as possible, free from stigma, well supported and socially included (Henwood and Downs, 2014).

Question: What other important points does the extract make? Readers might also want to research whether where they live would qualify for 'dementia-friendly' status.

## Prime Minister's challenge on dementia 2020

A second prime ministerial challenge followed in 2015 (Department of Health, 2015a). This summarised the progress that had been made since 2012 and contained a commitment to make England:

- the best country in the world for dementia care and support and for people with dementia, their carers and families to live and
- the best place in the world to undertake research into dementia and other neurodegenerative diseases.

The Implementation Plan that followed contained detailed steps that the government and other national bodies would take to improve the quality of life for people with dementia and their carers (Department of Health, 2016). These fell into four key themes:

- Risk reduction.
- Health and care.
- Dementia awareness and social action.
- Research.

2015 saw two important developments relevant to the social care workforce. *The Dementia Core Skills and Knowledge Framework* set out a broad curriculum and principles for training the social care workforce more generally (Skills for Care, 2015 – updated in 2018) and the *Manual for good social work practice: supporting adults who have dementia* (DH, 2015b) which is primarily a guide to practice for social workers supporting adults who have dementia and their carers. These, together with the messages contained in other relevant practice guidance, (e.g. *Dementia: assessment, management and support for people living with dementia and their carers*, NICE, 2018) will be discussed in Chapter 5.

## Dementia and adult safeguarding

Unfortunately, older adults with dementia are more likely to experience abuse and neglect than those without a diagnosis (Department of Health and Social Care, 2021). This includes all forms of abuse – psychological; physical; sexual; financial; emotional; neglect; self-neglect; organisational/institutional and domestic violence. There are many reasons why this is so. For example, having a cognitive impairment can make it easier to be taken advantage of or harmed and not be able to explain or communicate what is going on to others. Certain behaviours associated with forms of dementia such as becoming confused, aggressive, making repeated statements or incontinence can provoke abusive reactions in, already stressed, carers. The fact that sometimes dementia can cause hallucinations and delusions also means that attempts by the person to communicate abuse can be dismissed or rationalised as a symptom of the disease. Common reactions to abuse, such as withdrawal from communication, agitation, crying out and depression, can also be misinterpreted as symptoms of dementia rather than be seen as a response to being abused. These are some of the factors that suggest why people with dementia might be more at risk of abuse and why it can be harder to detect abuse directed towards people with dementia. The person is often either unable to recognise that they are being abused or they cannot communicate sufficiently clearly to explain what is happening (Alzheimer's Society, 2015). Responding effectively to suspicions or allegations of abuse in respect of someone with dementia can be a complex task. Consequently, it is important to understand the principles that underpin adult safeguarding policy.

The following sections are based on safeguarding in England. However, as frameworks differ across the four UK jurisdictions, readers from the other UK nations should check the details of their own national safeguarding guidance (Mac-Intyre, Stewart and McCusker, 2018). At the time of writing these were as follows but check for updates.

Northern Ireland: www.health-ni.gov.uk/articles/adult-safeguarding-prevention-and-protection-partnership/

Scotland: www.gov.scot/policies/social-care/adult-support-and-protection

Wales: www.gov.wales/safeguarding-guidance/

Guidance issued by the Department of Health (2010b) – *Nothing Ventured Nothing Gained* – made the point that decision making around risk and protection from risk needs to take into account the wellbeing and autonomy of the person with dementia, as well as their possible need for protection from physical or emotional harm. Safeguarding should be as much about looking at ways to empower people with dementia and promoting their quality of life as it is about removing or managing risks. The label of dementia should not mean that someone becomes the passive subject of overly protective and risk-averse decisions made by others. The approach expressed in the guidance is about balancing the need to protect a person considered as 'vulnerable' from harm with respecting their rights to independence and choice. The principles laid down in *Nothing Ventured Nothing Gained* echo the, now much-quoted, comments made by Lord Justice Munby, a judge who was President of the Family Division of the High Court of England and Wales. In his concluding comments on a case (not involving dementia) Munby stated:

> The emphasis must be on sensible risk appraisal, not striving to avoid all risk, whatever the price, but instead seeking a proper balance and being willing to tolerate manageable or acceptable risks as the price appropriately to be paid in order to achieve some other good – in particular to achieve the vital good of the elderly or vulnerable person's happiness. What good is it making someone safer if it merely makes them miserable?' Lord Justice Munby (2007).
>
> *(2007) cited in SCIE (2012: 28)*

Policy and practice in adult safeguarding in England is also informed by the *Making Safeguarding Personal* initiative (LGA, 2014). This development by the Local

Government Association (LGA) and the Association of Directors of Adults Social Services (ADASS) represents a coming together of the personalisation and adult safeguarding agendas in adult social care. *Making Safeguarding Personal* aims to ensure that safeguarding practice focuses on giving people choice when they are involved in safeguarding decisions and ensuring that, as far as possible, outcomes are in line with people's personal wishes.

A more recent development has been research-informed guidance derived from a collaboration between the Department of Health and Social Care and the University of Bath – *Supporting people living with dementia to be involved in adult safeguarding enquiries* (Department of Health and Social Care, 2021). More will be discussed about the practice guidance it provides in Chapter 5. However, the principles for practice outlined in the guidance are as follows:

The human rights of people living with dementia are protected in UK law through the Human Rights Act 1998 and the Convention on the Rights of Persons with Disabilities. FRIEDA principles can be used as a tool to remember how human rights laws should apply to people living with dementia. These principles focus on Fairness, Respect, Equality, Identity, Dignity and Autonomy.

Strengths-based approaches are a useful way of supporting the human rights of people who are living with dementia. Workers using this approach should identify things which the person is already successful at and seek to build on these. The approach also involves thinking about how issues of culture and diversity might have an impact on the decision in question.

Knowledge and understanding of relevant legislation and guidance is important for understanding how people living with dementia may be helped to partake in safeguarding enquiries. This includes knowledge of the Care Act 2014 and the related Care and Support Statutory Guidance, as well as the Mental Capacity Act 2005 and its Code of Practice and the Making Safeguarding Personal approach.

Supported decision-making frameworks can be used to assist people living with dementia to make decisions. Previous research has identified useful ways to assist decision making. These include listening to the person, asking the person about their preferences and choices in an open and non-challenging way, and providing the person with clear written information. Decision-making aids can be used to help people to structure such decisions (p. 6).

The references to 'FRIEDA' principles represent an updating of the original 'FREDA' principles which underpin international human rights treaties, the 1998 Human Rights Act and the Equality Act 2010. 'Identity' has subsequently been included partly because it links to the concept of 'personhood' (Butchard and Kinderman, 2019). The report explains that 'identity' in this context means: 'respect my intelligence, respect my skills and talents, respect my choices about how I want to live my life and let me live my life' (Department of Health and Social Care,

2021: 12). Therefore, policy on safeguarding people with living dementia highlights the need for practice to reflect, amongst other things, the human rights, choices, strengths, dignity and identity of the person with dementia. However, it also highlights the need for practice to take into account the key role played by carers, both as supporters of and advocates for people with dementia.

## The carers' agenda

Informal carers (family members, friends and neighbours) have long been recognised as mainstays of the adult social care system in the UK. In 2015, the economic value of the contribution made by carers in the UK was estimated at £132 billion per year, which was close to the total annual cost of health spending in the UK. The 2015 figure was 7% higher than for 2011. This is mostly because carers are providing more care in the day and over a longer period of years (Buckner and Yeandle, 2015). Because the role of informal carers in providing support for people living with dementia is so important, much government policy has been about both recognising and supporting the informal caring role. This includes providing respite, advice and other support services that promote carers' health and wellbeing (HM Government, 2008, 2010; NHS England, 2014; The Department of Health and Social Care, 2018a; LGA, 2018). In terms of financial support, the government first introduced the Carer's Allowance in 1976. This benefit has certain conditions attached to it but, at the time of writing is available for people over 16 years of age, who care for someone at least 35 hours a week and the person receives certain benefits such as Attendance Allowance or Personal Independence Payment.

Studies have shown that carers are not getting all the support to which they are entitled. For example, in 2020, around 1.1 million people in England were eligible to claim the Carer's Allowance, but only 780,000 people were receiving it (National Audit Office, 2021). More generally, many carers do not feel that they are recognised and valued. There are also gaps reported in provision across different areas as well as shortages of appropriate and timely advice (Newbronner et al., 2013). Some of these issues need to be addressed by better funding but others can be resolved by making sure that carers are properly informed of their rights.

## Policy context: key points

Social work practice with people living with dementia is informed by four major health and social care policy agendas: personalisation; adult safeguarding, caring for carers and, more specifically, the national dementia strategy. Anyone practising in this area of work needs to understand the drivers behind these agendas as well as the principles and values that inform them.

In terms of policy aimed directly at social work, the four countries of the UK have their own regulatory bodies for social work and social care. In England, all social work practice with people living with dementia and their carers needs to conform to the standards set out in the *Professional Capabilities Framework* (BASW, 2018) and *Professional Standards* (Social Work England, 2019). Social workers in their 'Assessed and Supported Year in Employment' (ASYEs) have been provided with additional guidance in the *Knowledge and Skills Statement for Social Workers in Adult Services* (Department of Health, 2015c). All of this practice guidance is informed by the policy agendas highlighted earlier. Practitioners in other countries need to check out the regulatory guidance relevant to their country, although in most cases, the core principles and underpinning values are the same. It is about taking an approach to practice that is person-centred, strengths-based, rights-based and socially inclusive.

## Legislative context

### The Human Rights Act 1998

As explained earlier, the WHO has called for a human rights-based approach to people living with dementia around the world. In the UK, the human rights of all citizens are underpinned by the Human Rights Act 1998 (HRA) that brought the European Convention on Human Rights (ECHR) into domestic law. Because of their cognitive and other impairments, people with dementia are at greater risk of having their human rights compromised, especially in the middle and latter stages of the disease. Human rights abuses do not just occur in institutional settings, they can occur when someone is cared for in their own home (Equality and Human Rights Commission, 2011). A guide that explains how the articles of the Human Rights Act 1998 translate into practice with people with dementia has been published by the British Institute of Human Rights (2016a). They place a particular focus on:

- Article 3 Right to be free from inhuman and degrading treatment.
- Article 5 Right to liberty.
- Article 8 Right to respect for private life, family life, and home.
- Article 14 Right to non-discrimination.

In practice, some rights, such as the right to liberty and the right to private and family life, are limited or qualified, meaning they can be restricted in certain circumstances. This would usually be in relation to safeguarding decisions, especially if the person is not considered to have capacity. Therefore, the Human Rights Act 1998 needs to be applied in conjunction with other relevant legislation such as the Care Act 2014, Mental Capacity Act 2005 and mental health legislation. The following case study is taken from another British Institute of Human Rights publication *Social Care Intervention and Human Rights: A practitioner's guide* (2016b). It illustrates how practitioners can use the HRA to protect the rights of people with dementia at critical moments in their lives.

## Case Study 3.3:   In real life: removing a person from their home unlawfully

Charlie, 91, has lived in his own home for 50 years. He is affected with dementia and has other health issues. A safeguarding alert is raised after a neighbour reported concerns about suspected financial abuse and his ability to selfcare. A capacity assessment concludes Charlie lacks capacity to make decisions about his care, residence and finances. Whilst residential care is investigated, a social worker receives a call from the neighbour requesting Charlie's urgent admission into residential care. The next morning Charlie is taken from his home. Although reluctant and distressed, his neighbour persuades him to go. Charlie is placed in a locked dementia unit against his will for 17 months. During this time, an urgent DoL authorisation is put in place, followed by a standard DoL authorisation, which expires. For several months, Charlie is detained without legal authorisation. The original capacity assessment contained no record of Charlie's wishes and feelings. Five other assessments take place; a social worker concludes Charlie doesn't have capacity to decide where to live, but a best interests assessor concludes Charlie does have capacity to decide this and recommends he is allowed home. Charlie's friend applies to the court challenging his care home placement. The court rules Charlie's placement was a breach of his right to liberty and private life. The local authority ignored the recommendation of the best interests assessor that the least restrictive option would be for Charlie to be supported to live at home. The local authority had also not taken seriously Charlie's consistently expressed wish to return home. Charlie returned home and the local authority had to pay damages for his unlawful detention. Being looked after by carers, Charlie is reported to be happy (adapted from British Institute of Human Rights, 2016b: 5).

'DoL', in the case study, refers to the Deprivation of Liberty Safeguards (DoLS) introduced in the Mental Capacity Act 2005. Standard and urgent DoLS 'authorisations' give managing authorities the power to deprive someone aged 18 or over of their liberty, in a hospital or care home, for the purpose of being given necessary care or treatment as long as the person lacks the capacity to consent to be there. From

April 2022, the DoLS system will be replaced by Liberty Protection Safeguards. See the section on the Mental Capacity Act for more details. The case study shows how the HRA can be used as a check and balance on decisions that restrict someone's liberty in a care setting.

## The Care Act 2014

In England, the legal framework for providing personalised care and support to adults with dementia who need it; for safeguarding adults in need of support and care who are considered at risk of abuse or neglect and for assessing the needs of carers and providing support where necessary, is set out in the Care Act 2014 (HM Government, 2014) and associated guidance (Department of Health, 2014). Social workers in adult services obviously need to be familiar with the Act in its entirety. However, some selected messages relevant to practice with dementia are highlighted here.

## Wellbeing

A key point about the Care Act 2014 was its focus on promoting wellbeing. The Act's concept of wellbeing is broad and wide-ranging – it encompasses more than just someone's health or their ability to manage activities of daily living. In the Act, it includes personal dignity; physical and mental health and emotional wellbeing; protection from abuse and neglect; control over day-to-day life (including care); participation in recreation; social and economic wellbeing; domestic, family and personal wellbeing and suitability of living accommodation (Braye and Preston-Shoot, 2020). The Care Act is underpinned by the basic assumptions that everyone's needs are different and individuals are best placed to judge their own individual wellbeing. It also advises that people should not just be considered as individuals with needs but in the context of their families and support networks. In other words, a whole family approach needs to be taken which means that consideration should be given to the impact of an individual's needs on the wellbeing of those who care for and support them.

## Preventing, reducing or delaying needs

Section 2 of the Care Act 2014 requires local and health authorities to operate on the principle of 'preventing, reducing or delaying needs'. It is about keeping people out of the formal health and social care system as long as possible by enabling them to be independent for as long as possible. Prevention can operate at three levels: primary; secondary and tertiary. Primary prevention is about taking action to reduce the incidence of disease and health problems within the population, either through universal measures that reduce lifestyle risks and their causes or by targeting high-risk groups. Secondary prevention is systematically detecting the early stages of the disease and intervening before full symptoms develop. Tertiary prevention means

> softening the impact of an ongoing illness or injury that has lasting effects. This is done by helping people manage long-term, often-complex health problems and injuries (e.g. chronic diseases, permanent impairments) in order to improve as much as possible their ability to function, their quality of life and their life expectancy.
>
> *(LGA, 2021)*

The social work role with people with dementia is more likely to be needed at the level of tertiary prevention. This is highlighted in *Care and support statutory guidance* (Department of Health, 2014) which is discussed in more detail in the section 'Care and support statutory guidance' which follows.

## Safeguarding

The Care Act 2014 incorporated the six principles of adult safeguarding set out by the Department of Health (2011b). These being:

1  Empowerment – people should be supported and encouraged to make their own decisions and give informed consent.
2  Prevention – it is better to take action before harm occurs.
3  Proportionality – pursue the least intrusive response appropriate to the risk presented.
4  Protection – adults should be supported to be free from harm and neglect.
5  Partnership – professionals should work *with* the person concerned to achieve the most effective solutions.
6  Accountability – it should be clear who is doing what and why.

## Carers

The Care Act 2014 recognises the role played by informal carers and considers that looking after the wellbeing of carers is as important as looking after the wellbeing of the person for whom they are caring. Consequently, if a carer appears to have needs from caring for a person eligible for care and support, the Act gives the carer the right to an assessment of needs. Local authorities have to consider the impact on the carer's wellbeing of performing their caring role. If the assessment shows that the carer's wellbeing is being significantly impacted by their caring role they are entitled to a service. This can be in the form of a personal budget and direct payment to pay for any services.

## Substantial difficulty and independent advocacy

Where people have 'substantial difficulty' in being involved in the key care and support processes of assessment, care and/or support planning, care reviews, safeguarding enquiries and safeguarding adult reviews, the Care Act 2014 states that reasonable steps must be taken to enable the person is fully involved. The Care Act 2014 defines four areas, in any one of which, a person might be found to have substantial difficulty. These are: *understanding* relevant information; *retaining information*; using or *weighing up* the information (as part of being involved in the key process); *communicating* their views, wishes and feelings. When deciding whether a person would experience substantial difficulty the Local Authority must have regard to:

a. Any health condition the person has;
b. Any learning difficulty the person has;
c. Any disability the person has;
d. The degree of complexity of the person's circumstances, whether in relation to their needs for Care and Support (or Support) or otherwise;
e. Where the assessment or planning function is the carrying out of an assessment (regardless of whether the person or carer has previously refused an assessment or not) and
f. Whether the person is experiencing, or at risk of, abuse or neglect.

By these criteria, most people with dementia will experience substantial difficulty as the disease progresses and come into one or more of the aforementioned categories.

In this context, Section 67 of the Act required local authorities to provide independent advocacy to facilitate the person's involvement in the care and support assessment, planning and review processes if they have 'substantial difficulty' and no other appropriate person is able to assist them. Section 68 of the Act states that the local authority must arrange, where appropriate, for an independent advocate to represent and support an adult who is the subject of a safeguarding enquiry or safeguarding adult review where the adult has 'substantial difficulty' in being involved in contributing to the process and where there is no other appropriate adult to assist.

As is evident from these brief summaries, the Care Act 2014 directs and mandates practice with people living with dementia and their carers that are personalised, promotes their wellbeing, is empowering, situates them in their wider social and family context and is socially inclusive. Its directions about substantial difficulty and advocacy underline an approach to practice that promotes the person's rights and their involvement in all parts of the care, support and safeguarding processes.

## Care and support statutory guidance

Statutory guidance to accompany the Care Act 2014 (Department of Health, 2014) is updated and amended from time to time to reflect regulatory changes, feedback from stakeholders and the care sector as well as court decisions. The most recent version can be found at: www.gov.uk/government/publications/care-act-statutory-guidance. The guidance provides more detail about how the principles and directions contained in the Care Act 2014 should be put into practice. It uses case studies to illustrate particular practice issues, including several that specifically reference dementia. In respect of people living with dementia, it provides a useful reference in making practice decisions around mental capacity, safeguarding and other important issues such as financial assessments and reviews of the care plan.

In paragraph 3.26, the guidance refers to the diagnosis of dementia as a 'trigger point' to which the response from the health and social care services should be to provide targeted information and advice. It underlines the importance of providing information about services that are both timely and at the right level to people with dementia and carers.

Paragraph 6.32 states that when there is concern about a person's capacity to make a specific decision, as a result of dementia, then an assessment of capacity should be carried out under the Mental Capacity Act 2005 (MCA). The guidance underlines how important it is for practitioners to be able to use the Care Act 2014 in conjunction with the Mental Capacity Act 2005 in cases that involve dementia.

## The Mental Capacity Act 2005

In England and Wales, the Mental Capacity Act 2005 (MCA) provides a legal framework to protect people in need of support and care and who lack capacity when critical decisions need to be made about their lives. Whereas the Care Act 2014 talks about assessing whether someone has 'substantial difficulty' in being involved in key care and support processes when someone is assessed to see whether they either have or lack capacity under the MCA, it is always in relation to a specific decision. Therefore, a determination of substantial difficulty for Care Act 2014 purposes is not a determination about mental capacity.

The five key principles of the MCA are:

1   Presumption of capacity: this means it is assumed that everyone has capacity until proved otherwise. A lack of capacity should not automatically be assumed simply based on a person's age, appearance, condition or behaviour. Therefore, a diagnosis of dementia does not automatically mean that someone lacks capacity.
2   Support to make a decision: this requires that all practical steps should be taken, to help the person make the decision themselves before treating them as unable to make the decision.
3   Ability to make unwise decisions: a person is not to be treated as unable to make a decision, merely because they make an unwise decision.
4   Best interest: if a decision is made (or an act done) on behalf of a person who does not have mental capacity, then it must be made (done) in their best interest.
5   Least restrictive: if a decision is made (or an act done) on behalf of a person who does not have mental capacity, it should ideally be the least restrictive option of the person's rights and freedoms. Other less restrictive options should be considered and applied if at all possible.

Because of the problems that cognitive deterioration can cause for people living with dementia in many areas of their lives, the MCA is a very important piece of legislation if and when people get to the point where they lack the mental capacity to make important decisions for themselves. This is an area of practice that raises some complex questions. For example, there is no legal definition of or simple answer to what constitutes a person's best interest. It comes down to professional judgement based on careful information gathering in relation to that specific individual. There is a procedure set out in Section 4 of the Mental Capacity Act (Department of Health, 2005a) which should be followed in such cases. An important additional safeguard brought in by the MCA is the creation of the Independent Mental Capacity Advocate (IMCA) role. This role is to support and represent the person in the decision-making process when they do not have appropriate family or friends to assist with important decisions.

All practitioners working with people under the Mental Capacity Act 2005 should refer to the *Mental Capacity Act Code of Practice* (Department of Constitutional Affairs, 2007) which provides practice guidance and explains what a practitioner's duties are in respect of the Act.

## The Court of Protection

In England and Wales, the Court of Protection deals with certain decisions or actions taken under the Mental Capacity Act 2005. For example, this could be deciding whether someone has the capacity to make a particular decision or whether a particular course of action is in their best interests. The Court of Protection can settle complex disagreements that cannot be settled even when an IMCA is involved. It also deals with challenges to DOLs authorisations and settles disputes about whether they are being used correctly.

Because it is a deteriorative condition, many people with dementia make plans for a time in the future when they can no longer make their own decisions about important matters. This commonly involves putting in place a Lasting Power of Attorney (LPA). This is a role introduced by the Mental Capacity Act 2005 in England and Wales. There are 'property and affairs' and 'health and welfare' LPAs. The property and financial affairs LPA would typically be concerned with decisions such as selling the person's property, managing their bank or building society account, paying bills or applying for welfare benefits. The health and welfare LPA would be involved with decisions regarding the person's health and social care including decisions about life-sustaining treatment. Unlike the property and affairs LPA, it can only be used once the person can no longer make their own decisions.

However, if no such arrangement has been made, and someone close to that person believes that they need to make decisions on their behalf, they need to apply to the Court of Protection to become their deputy. The Court has the power to remove an attorney or a deputy if they decide that the person is not making decisions or acting in their best interest. In some circumstances, the Court might appoint a professional such as a solicitor to be someone's deputy. In Scotland, people should contact the Office of the Public Guardian (Scotland) and in Northern Ireland the Office of Care and Protection in order to resolve these types of issues.

## Mental Health Acts 1983 and 2007

The Mental Health Act 1983 (as amended by the Mental Health Act 2007) gives health professionals (and AMHP trained social workers) the powers, to detain, assess and treat people with mental disorders in the interests of their health and safety or for public safety. For the purposes of the Mental Health Act, a diagnosis of dementia would be regarded as a mental disorder. The Act urges always taking the least restrictive option, so if a person with dementia is considered in need of hospital treatment and could be reasonably persuaded to be admitted as a voluntary patient, the Mental Health Act does not need to be used. However, at times, it is necessary to consider compulsory admission ('sectioning') when the person is not persuadable to seek hospital treatment and it appears that either they or someone else is at risk of harm if they do not receive it.

Under Section 2 of the Mental Health Act 1983, if the person with dementia was behaving in a way that posed a danger to their own health, or to the health of others, they could be detained in hospital for assessment by medical staff. The maximum amount of time someone can be detained under this section is 28 days. Two doctors need to agree that the section is necessary, one of them must be a mental health specialist (Section 12 approved), the other should be a doctor who knows the person well (often their GP). An application to detain someone under Section 2 also requires the signatures of an Approved Mental Health Professional (AMHP). The AMHP role could be performed by a social worker as long as they have completed the specialist training.

Section 3 is similar to Section 2 but can last for six months (or longer, if reviewed) and should only be used if a person needs treatment and refuses to accept it voluntarily. It is worth noting that if someone is detained under Section 3 of the Mental Health Act 1983 and it is decided that they need to be discharged to a care home, then Section 117 of the Act requires local authorities to provide free care home funding. Although this can be withdrawn if the NHS and local authority decide that the person's needs have changed.

Section 4 applies in emergency situations. Detention in a hospital must not last longer than 72 hours. One doctor and either an AMHP or the person's nearest relative can apply for a Section 4 order.

The 2007 Mental Health Act places a duty to make advocacy services available to detained patients. This Act created the Independent Mental Health Advocate (IMHA) role. An IMHA can be appointed regardless of someone has relatives or other informal advocates. Their role is to explain the detained person's rights and support the person to exercise those rights, for example, challenging their detention.

Although a diagnosis of dementia is considered to be a mental disorder for the purposes of mental health legislation, it is not usually the case that compulsory detention under the Mental Health Act is used to protect someone who is putting themselves at risk because of mild or moderate dementia. Sectioning is more likely to be considered when someone is in the latter stages of dementia and there is a real danger that they will harm themselves or others if that course of action was not taken. However, each case should be treated on its own merits depending on the needs of the person and what is in their best interests at that time.

## Summary

The policy and legislative context in which practice takes place with people with dementia mandate an approach that is person-centred, promotes wellbeing, rights, independence and choice, and focuses on the person's strengths wherever possible. However, because dementia is a deteriorative condition that can seriously someone's cognitive functioning making them at risk of harm, the legislation provides for proportionate interventions that can safeguard that person, even if it means restricting their choice, rights, and liberty. When someone no longer has the capacity to make informed decisions, the key question for decision-makers is to ask 'what is in that person's best interests'? Checks and balances through, for example, the use of independent advocacy have been introduced to ensure that any interventions are proportionate and the least restrictive option is always taken. The need to recognise and support the role of informal carers is a major plank of all policy and legislation in respect of working with dementia.

## Further reading

Braye, S. and Preston-Shoot, M. (Eds). (2020). *The Care Act 2014: Wellbeing in Practice*. London: Sage.
    This book is not specifically about dementia practice. However, its contributors provide a useful guide for social work practitioners, not only on to how to navigate the Care Act 2014, Mental Capacity Act 2005 and other relevant legislation but they also discuss relevant debates and issues that impact on dementia practice.
MacIntyre, G., Stewart, A. and McCusker, P. (Eds). (2018). *Safeguarding Adults*. Basingstoke: Palgrave.
    This book covers all aspects of adult safeguarding. It is recommended here because it covers legislation and policy across all four UK jurisdictions.

# 4
# APPROACHES TO DEMENTIA CARE

By the end of this chapter, you should have an understanding of:

- Bio-medical, person-centred and rights-based approaches to dementia care.
- The role of palliative care and ACP in dementia care.

## Introduction

Responses to dementia by medical, health, social care and other services have evolved over time. The different professions have tended to draw upon differing conceptual frameworks, knowledge bases and professional philosophies in determining what their role is, what their objectives should be and what services and treatments should be provided to people living with dementia. Approaches have developed in response to new medical knowledge and changing ideas within the health professions but also from the influence of other disciplines such as psychology and sociology. In recent decades, philosophical concepts such as 'personhood', identity and human rights, as well as the desire to include the lived experiences of people with dementia have all made a significant impact on models of treatment and care. Therefore, over time, different approaches to dementia care have emerged and evolved. Some have built on what has gone before, whilst others have challenged prevailing ideas.

This chapter focuses on broad approaches that have been widely adopted in the UK and in many countries around the world, such as Kitwood's 'person-centred' approach (Kitwood, 1997) and the approaches that it has inspired, such as the VIPS Framework© (Brooker, 2007). It will also examine approaches that incorporate ideas about human rights and the social model of disability. Finally, the chapter discusses the important role that palliative care can play for people with dementia

DOI: 10.4324/9781003191667-5

and their caregivers as the disease progresses. Part of this involves the consideration of advance care planning and matters related to end-of-life care.

Throughout the chapter, the terms 'model' and 'approach' will be used almost interchangeably. However, it is acknowledged that these are only approximations. When either term is used it refers to the broad conceptual framework and knowledge base that informs practice with people with dementia and, as a consequence, the principles and values upon which services and interventions are delivered. In Chapter 1, it was explained that approaches to dementia are still largely dominated by the 'bio-medical model'. Therefore, the chapter begins with a critical discussion of this approach to dementia care.

## Bio-medical model

The bio-medical approach in medicine generally focuses on the molecular biology of diseases and understanding the chemical and physical reasons for organic abnormalities. The core of the bio-medical approach is founded on the principle that health problems have biological or physical causes and that they are treatable with biological or physical methods.

Because the bio-medical model is founded on medical science it means that decisions about treatment are primarily in the hands of the 'experts' – typically medical professionals. This can leave the person with the disease (the 'patient' in medical discourse) feeling that they have little control or power over what course their treatment and care should take.

As explained in Chapter 1, the bio-medical approach to dementia perceives it primarily as a pathological condition to be diagnosed and treated medically. Cheston and Bender (1999) refer to the bio-medical approach as the 'organic' model in the sense that it focuses primarily on understanding the workings of the brain as the organ of the body which controls all our important physical and mental functions.

It is a common misunderstanding that all doctors and health professionals adopt a narrow bio-medical approach to dementia in their practice. In reality, the various health professions will often incorporate a broader understanding of the presenting problem and clinical attention is given to the psychological, environmental and other domains of human life (Farre and Rapley, 2017). Therefore, to some extent, the bio-medical model in its purest and narrowest form could be said to exist as an 'oppositional construct' or stereotype, with which to illuminate and argue for other approaches (Innes and Manthorpe, 2012). That said, the bio-medical approach to dementia remains dominant in dementia care for various reasons. These are partly because of the traditional power of the medical profession, partly because it is regarded as 'properly' scientific and 'evidence-based' and also because many people put their faith in the fact that, this approach will, one day, find a cure.

The reason for starting with the bio-medical approach to dementia is, first, because, as stated, it still holds sway over the medical and many other professions in health and social care and, for different reasons, provides a point of reference and a way of understanding dementia that is comprehensible to many people with the disease and their carers (Estes and Binney, 1989; Parker, 2001). As explained in Chapter 1, the bio-medical discourse has become the 'natural' discourse of dementia. For example, it informs NHS guidance and many other sources of reputable information that people use. Second, understanding the bio-medical approach helps understand why more person-centred approaches to dementia have developed in recent decades. This has happened primarily as a rejection of the impact the bio-medical approach has had on the way that people with dementia are viewed and, as a consequence, services are organised and delivered. Amongst other things, the narrow bio-medical approach has been criticised for ignoring social, environmental and cultural factors and disregarding the person's subjective experience of living with the disease (Innes and Manthorpe, 2012).

In 1977, George Engel, an American Professor of Psychiatry and Medicine, articulated what he believed was wrong with the bio-medical approach to psychiatry in general:

> The dominant model of disease today is biomedical, with molecular biology its basic scientific discipline. It assumes disease to be fully accounted for by deviations from the norm of measurable biological (somatic) variables. It leaves no room within its framework for the social, psychological, and behavioral dimensions of illness. The biomedical model not only requires that disease be dealt with as an entity independent of social behavior, it also demands that behavioral aberrations be explained on the basis of disordered somatic (biochemical or neurophysiological) processes. Thus the biomedical model embraces both reductionism, the philosophic view that complex phenomena are ultimately derived from a single primary principle, and mind-body dualism the doctrine that separates the mental from the somatic.
>
> *(Engel, 1977: 130)*

It is interesting to see that this critique came from within psychiatry, which somewhat undermines the belief that all psychiatrists are interested only in biomedicine. As Engel says, the bio-medical model 'leaves no room within its framework for the social, psychological, and behavioral dimensions of illness'. He was calling for psychiatrists to take a much more holistic view of the human subject and of mental illness. In terms of dementia specifically, Lyman (1989) made a similar critique, stating that:

> the biomedical view of dementia is narrow, limited, and sometimes distorted in its ignorance of social forces that affect the definition, production, and progression of dementia.
>
> *(1989: 600)*

Lyman criticised the bio-medical model for advancing the view that dementia progresses in defined and predictable stages of decline. She argues that acceptance of this view paves the way for caregivers to consider that some form of institutionalisation must be an inevitable destination for the person with dementia. However, in one landmark study, Gubrium (1987) found, in his close analysis of people with Alzheimer's disease, that their disease did not necessarily follow the ordered sequence of stages that bio-medical texts described and predicted. There was significant variation between different individuals. The important point for health and social care professionals to take from this is not to accept uncritically the view that a diagnosis of dementia involves a staged decline, leading inevitably to the person needing institutional care. To do so is overly deterministic and closes off the possibility of other, more person-centred and creative options.

In summary, the bio-medical approach to dementia is criticised for its reductionism, putting too much emphasis on understanding the effects of organic functioning whilst ignoring social, psychological and other factors that shape the individual experience of living with dementia (Kitwood and Bredin, 1992). By explaining dementia as a disease of progressive stages of deterioration, the model is criticised for generalising or homogenising the condition, when this might not be the case for all individuals living with it (Cheston and Bender, 1999). The reductionism of the bio-medical approach has implications for how people are cared for once a diagnosis has been made. Cheston and Bender (1999) argue that there is too much emphasis placed on assessment, especially on the assessment of the person's memory, which is not always accurate and can be an upsetting experience in itself. Other than regular assessments, the main preoccupations of the bio-medical model are symptom management and the regulation of behaviour (Vernooij-Dassen et al., 2019). Based on the assumption that mental deterioration will render the person incapable of deciding or communicating for themselves, the focus of care regimes based on a bio-medical approach can easily tend to focus on keeping the person safe from harm and maintaining their personal hygiene but paying little or no regard to their social, psychological, spiritual or sexual needs (Harding and Palfrey, 1997; Archibald, 2004). At its most reductive, the bio-medical model predicts that the impact of the disease gets steadily and relentlessly worse until the 'person' living with it becomes 'lost' completely. The determinism of this view is criticised because it can lead to pre-programmed and unimaginative thinking about care options that focus on bodily maintenance and personal care and, in some ways, become a self-fulfilling prophecy. Adams and Bartlett (2003) suggest that the depersonalising side effects of the bio-medical approach not only constitutes the person as more of an object to be 'done to', the person is also placed at greater risk from abusive, oppressive and discriminatory practices from health and social care workers as a consequence.

Thus far, the discussion has highlighted several of the main criticisms of the bio-medical model. However, it needs to be acknowledged that bio-medicine has made important contributions to the understanding of dementia. For a start, in confirming that dementia is a pathological condition with organic causation, the bio-medical model countered long-held ageist assumptions that going 'senile' was a normal part of getting older (Lyman, 1989). Bio-medical research has led to a better understanding of brain functioning and the ageing brain generally (Winblad et al., 2016). It has been able to distinguish between different types of dementia, which means that the person's experiences can be better understood and treatments can be better targeted. Despite the fact that no cure has been found for any type of dementia yet, bio-medical science provides hope that, someday, one will be found. It has added to the scientific evidence base around medicines and other treatments for dementia which helps improve their effectiveness. The fact is that neither prevention in the future nor an effective cure will be possible without bio-medical research (Lyman, 1989). Diagnosis can prove to be very useful for people with dementia and their carers, allowing them to make sense of what is happening to them. The ongoing contribution of bio-medicine in understanding and treating various forms of dementia should not be dismissed.

## Beyond the bio-medical model: bio-psycho-social, person-centred and rights approaches

It was discussed earlier how George Engel argued that the traditional bio-medical approach to mental illness was fundamentally limited in its scope. Instead, Engel argued for a 'new medical model' – a bio-psycho-social model of psychiatry (Engel, 1977). He was interested in understanding the interplay of the 'bio' (the biological understanding of the disease); the 'psycho' (the person's inner world, their thoughts, emotions and feelings) and the 'socio' (the person in their social or sociological context). Bio-psycho-social approaches to dementia began to develop from the 1980s onwards, gaining prominence through the work of the social psychologist Tom Kitwood who is probably the person most associated with laying the foundations for 'person-centred' approaches to dementia care (Sabat, 2014).

### Person-centred

What 'person-centred' means both theoretically and in practice is contested. It can mean different things to different people in different contexts and therefore providing a simple definition is not straightforward (Brooker, 2007). An important question to consider would be 'what or who exactly is it that the bio-medical approach to dementia is not taking into consideration?' Now, at first glance, this might look like a perfectly straightforward question to answer. However, when examined more closely, it raises complex, philosophical questions about the nature of 'the self', what it is that makes us who we are and what it is to be a human being. This line of questioning not only takes us into philosophical but also spiritual territory. These questions are complex and will certainly not be resolved here. However, they are raised to make the point that the shift towards person-centred approaches in dementia care is, on one level, about changing practices and, perhaps more important, changing cultures (Dewing and McCormack, 2016). However, on another, deeper level, it is important to understand or, at least, give thought to the philosophical underpinning of person-centred approaches to practice.

Tom Kitwood was not a psychiatrist and came relatively late to dementia studies. Ordained as a priest, he was also qualified in organic chemistry and social
psychology. He was later to found and become the leader of the Bradford University Dementia Group (Woods, 1999). Similar to Gubrium, Kitwood's ideas about
dementia care were developed from observing care practices at close quarters in
the 1980s. Apart from his background in Christian theology, he was influenced
by the writings of contemporaries such as Sabat and Harré (1992) and Post (2000)
and particularly by the philosopher Martin Buber (1937) and humanist psychologist Carl Rogers (1961). From these foundations, Kitwood developed his ideas
about 'personhood' which, he argued, were central to a person-centred approach
to dementia care.

In 1989, Kitwood, with a fellow member of Bradford Dementia Research
Group, Kathleen Bredin, published a seminal paper in which they wrote:

> The psychiatry of old age has had an overwhelming tendency to make the
> brain rather than the personhood of the dementia sufferer its central focus of
> attention; the inquiry has been technical rather than personal. This has been
> very useful for medical-scientific research, but it has delivered almost no val-
> uable theoretical insight into the practicalities of care. Behind this lies the fact
> that both psychiatry and clinical psychology have been extremely reluctant to
> articulate and implement a clear concept of the human subject, preferring to
> work even at a clinical level with regularities among fairly simple observables.
> *(Kitwood and Bredin, 1992: 270)*

Therefore, as Kitwood (1997) was to write later, 'our frame of reference should no
longer be person-with DEMENTIA, but PERSON-with dementia' [sic] (p. 7).
Kitwood was making the point that by focusing on the malfunctioning brain, the
person (whose brain it is) gets lost. The human subject (the person) should always
come first. Kitwood did not deny that neurological impairment impacted on the
person, but he argued that good dementia care required understanding how the
person's neurological impairment interacted with their individual psychology,
their social context, their sense of self and spirituality. This shifted the attention to
the way someone's 'personhood' could either be preserved or threatened by their
social-psychological environment. For Kitwood, communication and relationships
were critical components of this environment. Much of his work was about how
to utilise these components in order to promote the wellbeing of people living
with dementia.

## Personhood

What constitutes or defines personhood raises some complex, philosophical questions and Kitwood has been criticised for failing to define this concept sufficiently
clearly to make it possible to verify empirically (Higgs and Gilleard, 2016). However, through Kitwood's focus on the person, he makes several important points

that are pertinent to dementia care. Perhaps most illuminating about what defines personhood for Kitwood is his discussion about the difference between 'I Thou' and 'I It' modes of relating.

## I Thou and I It modes

Kitwood's ideas about personhood are tied to how people relate to each other. Drawing on Buber's work, Kitwood says that people can address each other in an 'I It' mode or an 'I Thou' mode. 'I It' is a mode of relating to others that is impersonal, detached and gives very little of yourself to the other. As a consequence, they are less of a person in that interaction and more of an object. Kitwood (1997) says that relationships of the I-It kind are basically instrumental and 'can never rise beyond the banal or trivial' (p. 10). Consumer transactions often take place with both people using 'I It' mode. On the other hand, Kitwood (quoting Buber) says that 'to be a person is to be addressed as Thou' (ibid.). The 'I Thou' mode means relating to someone with respect, spontaneity and a willingness to open yourself up to the other person. In this mode of interaction, personhood is both expressed and validated. For Kitwood, this form of relationship is therefore not merely instrumental but transcendental. He believed that the I Thou mode has both ethical and spiritual dimensions because it recognises the other's worth and standing as a human being. Therefore, according to Kitwood, personhood arises from social relationships – specifically from relationships between 'Thous'.

This represents something of necessary over simplification of what Kitwood says in full about the 'I Thou' mode and its relationship to personhood, partly because he starts to lose some philosophical coherence the more he explores the subject (Greenwood, 1998; Dewing, 2008; Higgs and Gilleard, 2016). However, if we assume that personhood equates to what we might call someone's sense of self or their identity (Butchard and Kinderman, 2019), the basic idea provides important points to consider for health and social care professionals working with dementia. They are that dementia does not inevitably destroy someone's personhood over time. If you want to find and relate to the person inside you need to search for them. This will not happen if you don't think there is anyone or anything there. However, personhood *is* threatened and probably lost by being related to by 'I It' modes of communication and interaction. 'I Thou' modes of relating can preserve someone's personhood by being respectful, self-disclosing and open – giving of oneself. Quality of communication is crucial but so is the belief that someone's personhood endures as their dementia progresses.

## Malignant social psychology and positive person work

Kitwood (1997) argued that people with dementia have basic psychological needs that need to be met if their personhood is to be preserved and their physical and emotional wellbeing promoted. These are the need for comfort, attachment, inclusion, occupation and identity. His research revealed a 'dark picture' whereby care regimes were generally failing to meet most, if not all, of these needs. Kitwood developed the idea of 'malignant social psychology' from his observations of the way staff treated people with dementia in care settings. It links closely to the idea that the quality of communication and social relationships can either validate or threaten someone's personhood. Kitwood illustrates this concept with a grotesque vignette drawn from real life which depicts a group of people with dementia enduring a series of depersonalising and dehumanising indignities, whilst supposedly in the 'care' of staff in an unnamed setting. The example contains multiple examples of what Kitwood called 'personal detractions'. These are behaviours by the staff that demeaned and humiliated the people they were meant to be caring for and, in so doing, undermined their personhood. Kitwood's research led him to contend that such harmful practices were far from untypical in dementia care settings and referred to them as a form of 'malignant social psychology' that had become part of the culture of dementia care at that time (Kitwood, 1997). Malignant social psychology exacerbates the negative impact that the actual disease itself has on a person. Not only must they face the struggle of losing cognitive functions, but people living with dementia are also made to feel worthless by the 'malignant' actions and attitudes of others.

On the other hand, Kitwood observed actions and behaviours by staff that enhanced the personhood of those for whom they were caring and promoted their wellbeing. Kitwood calls these 'positive events'. From these Kitwood (1997) developed the idea of 'positive person work' which can help meet the emotional needs of people living with dementia and thus enhance their psychological wellbeing and preserve their personhood.

## Malignant social psychology – personal detractions

By 1997, Kitwood had formulated a list of 17 types of personal detractions. These are provided here. A basic explanation about what they mean has been added:

1 Treachery. Deceiving or manipulating a person into doing what you want them to do. An example might be telling someone that they are going for a drive out to get some fresh air when they are actually being taken to see the doctor.
2 Disempowerment. Stopping someone from doing something or failing to provide the necessary support to enable them to do something. Making someone feel as if they have no control over their lives.
3 Infantilisation. As it says, basically treating someone like a child. Being patronising.
4 Intimidation. Coercing someone to do something by threatening them in some way.
5 Labelling. Using a label such as their diagnosis to refer to them rather than treat them as an individual, for example, He's 'fronto-temporal'. Describing someone as 'challenging', 'difficult' or a 'bit of a wanderer' is also labelling and robs that person of their individuality.

6   Stigmatisation. Stereotyping someone in such a way that they are regarded as inferior to and treated worse than others. This will often cause them to feel worse about themselves. This often happens in conjunction with labelling.

7   Outpacing. Knowingly putting someone under unnecessary pressure to do things more rapidly than they are able. For example, talking too fast, walking too fast or rushing them in the toilet. It brings attention to and underlines their deficits and what they cannot do.

8   Invalidation. Not given someone's actions, experiences and feelings the recognition they deserve.

9   Banishment. Not only asking or telling someone to move somewhere else physically but also excluding them psychologically. Isolating someone for 'difficult' behaviour for which they cannot be held responsible.

10   Objectification. Treating someone simply as the body they inhabit to be cleaned, fed and 'done to'. This might be carelessly pushing and pulling someone around to dress them or to help them out of bed or simply shoving a spoonful of food in their mouths at dinner time. It might also be talking about them in their presence as if they cannot hear or are not aware of being talked about.

11   Ignoring. As it says, 'blanking' the person as if they do not exist. Zoning someone out even if it is obvious that they are trying to get attention.

12   Imposition. Getting someone to do something that they would not necessarily want to do if they were able to resist. For example, wait in a wheelchair in a corridor whilst other jobs are attended to.

13   Withholding. Being aware that someone wants or needs something but deliberately not giving it to them. Making them wait for no reason. This could apply equally to emotional withholding.

14   Accusation. Accusing somebody of doing or saying something as if they had no cognitive impairment, whilst knowing that their impairment means they do not realise they are doing it. Examples might include 'Why have you come to the office, you know you shouldn't be here'? or 'Look at the mess in this bed. I suppose I have to clear that up when I've got enough to do already!'.

15   Disruption. Cutting across someone whilst they are in the process of saying or doing something in a way that upsets them because they lose the thread of what they were thinking or saying. Leaving someone needlessly confused or frustrated.

16   Mockery. Making fun of someone's confusion or other difficulties – especially in front of others.

17   Disparagement. Undermining someone's sense of self-worth by criticising them unnecessarily.

It is evident from the list that there are overlaps between the detractions and the brief glossary that I have given to each is for illustrative purposes. It does not claim to be definitive or comprehensive. There can often be a context when these things happen, which Kitwood recognised, such as stressful working conditions, staff shortages and so on. However, Kitwood argued that care staff had a choice in how to relate to people in their care and the moral choice was to avoid using any type of personal detraction.

## Activity 4.1: Elderly Care Exposed

This activity involves tracking down, via YouTube or some other means, the BBC Panorama programme first broadcast on 30 April 2014 called 'Behind Closed Doors: Elderly Care Exposed'. It is an exposé using hidden camera techniques of abusive care practices in a care home where many of the residents had some form of dementia.

- Use Kitwood's list of personal detractions to identify the ways in which the resident's personhood is denied and their dignity as human beings disregarded.
- Reflect on how this was able to happen a good decade or so after Kitwood identified such abuses.
- Whilst the home in question might not be typical of all care homes, think how and why personal detractions might still happen in less obviously abusive but more subtle ways in other settings.

Whilst some of the practice observed in the programme might not be considered typical of all care homes, the programme illustrates well the vulnerability of people in such situations and how reliant they are on care from others to have their needs met and to lead their lives as best as possible. Unfortunately, the programme underlines that living with dementia is challenging enough, but living with dementia in an environment of malign social psychology makes the impact of having the disease much worse.

It is important to point out that Kitwood's personal detractions are not always what might be formally classifiable as abuse or safeguarding concerns. They could be more accurately described as poor quality care. Examples include a care worker casually wheeling someone out of the room without explaining what was happening to them or ignoring what they are trying to say whilst having a conversation with another worker or talking on their phone to a friend whilst escorting a person on a walk outside. Unfortunately, such thoughtless and disrespectful practices are not uncommon in many care situations. They diminish not only the person being cared for, but also the person who is supposed to be providing the care.

### *Positive person work*

Kitwood argued that through 'positive person work' caregivers could meet the psychological needs of people with dementia and, consequently, enhance their personhood. Kitwood's 12 categories of positive person work are:

1 Recognition
2 Negotiation
3 Collaboration
4 Play
5 Timalation

6   Celebration
7   Relaxation
8   Validation
9   Holding
10   Facilitation
11   Creation
12   Giving

*(Kitwood, 1997: 119–120)*

As with the personal detractions, the meaning of many of these practices is largely self-evident. All of them involve a high degree of engagement with the person and connecting with them in ways that allow not only their personhood to be preserved but enhanced if possible. 'Timalation' refers to sensual and tactile interactions and practices that stimulate the senses such as aromatherapy or massage. 'Validation' requires a high degree of empathy. It is not just about recognising a person's worth, but also about giving validity to the reality of their experiences, which might well include hallucinative or delusional content and might not be real for us but is for them. 'Holding' is not necessarily holding someone physically although this can comforting when done appropriately. It more refers to holding someone emotionally and making them feel safe and secure. 'Creation' refers to the fact that using play and other creative activities such as art, singing or gardening with someone who has problems communicating can often enable them to express themselves better and give them more pleasure than engaging them in conversation. 'Giving' refers back to the 'I Thou' mode of relating and also requires a high degree of empathy. It means being prepared to give something of oneself self to the person with dementia and not just hiding behind a role. It can also mean being warm and generous in how any gifts given to you from the person are received. Kitwood therefore not only highlighted damaging care practices but also provided care workers with a set of tools with which to enhance the personhood of those with whom they work. Somewhat controversially, Kitwood proposed the possibility of 'rementia', where, with enough positive person work, the effects of someone's dementia are reversed and lost functions restored. However, there is no reliable evidence base for this at the moment.

## Dementia Care Mapping

Building on the idea of malign social psychology and the importance of the psychosocial environment in care, Kitwood developed Dementia Care Mapping (DCM). DCM is a form of structured observation used in dementia care settings both to measure and improve person-centred care. A team of non-participant observers (mappers) watch interactions between the care staff and those for whom they are caring over a period of hours. They note both positive care actions (the personal enhancers) that improve someone's wellbeing and negative care actions (the personal detractions) that decrease wellbeing or create ill-being (Bradford Dementia

Group, 2005). The results are used to improve practice and help create a more enabling culture. Some studies have found that DCM is not always effective nor is it possible to implement it in the way it was designed for various reasons, including organisational and other contextual factors (Griffiths et al., 2019; Surr et al., 2020). This means that DCM should not necessarily be seen as a silver bullet. It is not always possible to change care cultures fundamentally. However, Brooker (2005) concluded that 'DCM holds a unique position in relation to quality of life in dementia care, being both an evaluative instrument and as a vehicle for practice development in person-centered care (p. 17)'.

Taken together, the concepts of malignant social psychology, positive person work and DCM have two obvious implications for social work practice. They underline the importance of respectful, person-centred communication and positive, affirmative interactions in social workers' professional relationships with people living with dementia. However, they also provide social workers with a framework with which to assess the quality of care in settings in which they might place or have already placed people living with dementia. People with dementia should not be placed nor should have to live in an environment of malign social psychology. The tools and concepts developed by Kitwood, therefore, provide a framework and a language with which to assess care settings and to advocate for change where necessary. More will be discussed on the social work role in this respect in Chapter 5.

### Critiques and refinements of Kitwood

Most would agree that Tom Kitwood played a huge part in changing the culture of dementia care from a narrowly bio-medical organic approach to a much more person-centred approach (Kitwood and Brooker, 2019). As highlighted earlier, some have questioned the coherence of Kitwood's conceptualisation of personhood (Greenwood, 1998; Dewing, 2008; Higgs and Gilleard, 2016). Also, Mac-Rae (2009) suggested that people with dementia can preserve their personhood themselves, despite the particular psycho-social environment in which they find themselves, by tapping into their own past biographical experiences and memories. Meanwhile, Kontos (2005) argued that, whilst Kitwood's view of personhood included the psycho-social components of the self, it took insufficient account of the corporeal element that makes us who we are and contributes towards our sense of self. She proposed that 'selfhood emanates from the body's power of natural expression' (p. 561) and argued that people's 'embodied selfhood' should be at the core of dementia care. This, it should be noted, does not mean just attending to the care of the person's body, it means understanding how the person is using their body to express themselves. This view challenges the idea that, as dementia progresses, the 'person' leaves the body, simply leaving a corporeal shell. Kontos would argue that, on the contrary, the embodied self is the person. It is their prime mode of being in the world. Others have also argued that Kitwood's person-centred approach does not encapsulate notions of citizenship, embodiment and other dimensions of the experience of living with dementia (Hampson and Morris, 2016).

Like many others, Davis (2004) praises Kitwood's humane approach to dementia care but criticises the idea that someone's personhood can be maintained even in its very advanced stages. He says that buying into this idea 'amounts to the acceptance of a false sense that selfhood is resistant even to dementia-disease' (p. 377). Davis says that if it is held to be true that someone's personhood endures, but their carers do not, in all honesty, recognise the person they once knew, it suggests they have not worked hard enough at the relationship. This, Davis argues, most likely adds a sense of guilt to the feelings of loss they would already be experiencing. He concludes by calling for 'greater honesty in determining the violence that dementia does to the substance of the person and absolve those closest relations of the guilt of overseeing this decline' (p. 377). In many ways, this is a head-on challenge to the idea that someone's personhood endures throughout the progression of the disease, at least in ways that are recognisable to those who know them. It illustrates some of the philosophical complexities underpinning person-centred approaches.

Much of the work developing and refining Kitwood's approach to dementia care has come from the nursing profession and from gerontological nursing in particular (McCormack, 2004). In a review of the literature, McCormack (2004) identified five different models of person-centred care that have followed Kitwood. These were McCormack's own model, which he called the 'Authentic Consciousness Framework'; 'Positive person work' (Packer, 2003); the 'Senses Framework' (Nolan, Davies and Grant, 2001); 'Skilled companionship' (Titchen, 2001) and 'The Burford Nursing Development Unit (BNDU) model of nursing' (Johns, 1994).

The models McCormack identifies are not all designed specifically with dementia in mind. However, each model develops a dimension to caring for people with dementia that either Kitwood did not include or develops an idea further. For example, a key focus of 'skilled companionship' is building a close, empathetic relationship in which the professional (a nurse in Titchen's case) is prepared to express their own vulnerability (Titchen, 2001). The requirement that the professional should be prepared to be emotionally engaged and to give of themselves is very much akin to what Kitwood (1997) identifies as 'giving' in positive person work. However, Nolan, Davies and Grant (2001) in developing the 'Senses Framework' argue for more of a systemic approach than Kitwood. In the 'Senses Framework', everybody involved with the person's care (the person, their family carers and care staff) need a 'sense' of: security; continuity, belonging, purpose, achievement and significance in order to function effectively. Nolan, Davies and Grant (2001), therefore, stress the importance of understanding the interdependencies between the person with dementia, their family caregivers and paid care professionals in providing care that is person-centred but recognises that that person is part of a broader support system.

McCormack concludes that the recurring patterns and themes in relation to all these models are:

> knowing the person (of the patient and nurse), values, biography, relationships, seeing beyond the immediate needs and authenticity.
>
> *(p. 36)*

This suggests that, in practice, it is possible to skirt around some of the knottier philosophical questions about personhood and focus on 'knowing the person', primarily through building respectful, empathetic and honest relationships both with the individual in question and significant others around them.

## Person-focused approach

Cheston and Bender (1999) take exception to the term 'person-centred' partly because of its associations with Rogerian counselling and, instead, explain that their own approach is 'person-focused'. This is also because they want to draw attention to the actual process of bringing someone with dementia into focus as a person. According to Cheston and Bender (1999: 112) features of the person-focused approach to dementia are:

1   Dementia needs to be understood as an interaction between psychosocial and neurological influences.
2   The main focus of dementia care must be on the person living with the illness, alongside an awareness of the needs of carers.
3   Dementia is a terrifying ordeal which creates an enormous sense of insecurity within individuals and generates an emotional reaction.
4   The impact of the process of dementia is also experienced in terms of a threat to the person's view of themselves as a coherent entity.
5   The threat to a person's identity that is posed by dementia precipitates a range of behaviours whose function is to assert the individual's identity.
6   In order to understand the behaviour of a person living with dementia, we also need to understand their fears and the way in which they assert their own identity.
7   Without such an understanding of the emotional and identity needs of dementia sufferers we are liable to misinterpret the behaviour that arises when these needs are not met as resulting from neurological damage.
8   We need to understand how a person with dementia is valued in their society and the effects – economic and social – of that valuation.
9   Once we have begun to understand the emotional, identity and social frameworks within which a dementia sufferer lives, then we can begin to develop effective, life-enhancing forms of help.

As is evident, there is much overlap between taking a person-centred and person-focused approach both in principle and practice. Cheston and Bender make a valid point about the associations of 'person-centred' with counselling, but person-centred is the phrase that has gained more traction in the world of dementia care.

## Psychological therapies

Around about the time Kitwood was developing his ideas, clinical psychologists were also developing different therapeutic interventions designed to improve the mental health of people living with dementia. The most well known are probably reality orientation (RO) (Rimmer, 1982; Holden and Woods, 1988), reminiscence therapy (Norris, 1986), resolution therapy (Stokes and Goudie, 1990) and validation therapy (Feil, 1993). (See also the section on Memory Clinics in Chapter 6.)

RO is an approach where the focus is to improve the cognitive functioning of someone with dementia by orientating them back to the reality of the 'here and now'. This might involve using the person's name often when talking to them and incorporating repeated references to current events (in the person's life and in the outside world in general) into interactions with the person. The physical environment in a care home using RO techniques might use signage to help the person orientate themselves in terms of the time, date, locations and current surroundings. So, for example, each day the staff will change the signs throughout the home to show that day's date, the weather and so on. Advocates of RO claim that it can improve someone's cognitive abilities. However, when carried out without empathy, this approach has been criticised for being inappropriately challenging for people with dementia. At its worst, it is argued that the use of RO, without proper consideration of the person's individual situation, can cause unnecessary distress, resurrect grief responses and create frustration on both sides.

Partly over concerns about how it has been used in practice, RO has seen a decline in popularity in recent times. Approaches such as resolution therapy and validation therapy have been introduced as effective ways of helping people with dementia to make sense of what has been happening to them whilst taking better account of their emotions and perceptions − their individual realities. These approaches aim to both understand and work with the subjective reality of the person rather than dismiss or try to correct it. Therefore, validation therapy involves communicating with a person with dementia by respecting their thoughts and feelings in whatever time or place or context is real to the person at the time, even though it might not correspond to what we might consider to be the present reality (Feil, 1993).

Resolution therapy is a way of working with people with dementia where the aim is to uncover the hidden meanings and feelings that underly that person's confused verbal and behaviour. It is argued that, however confused they might seem, these behaviours have a meaning and relevance to the person. By listening to and observing the person empathetically, it can be possible to gain an idea of what the meaning behind certain behaviours is. From this, with a better understanding of the person's feelings and of how they are seeing the world, comes the possibility of improving their situation and helping them make better sense of their situation and finding some psychological comfort in the process (Stokes and Goudie, 1990).

Reminiscence therapy in dementia care can take a variety of forms (Norris, 1986). However, basically, it involves focusing on someone's past life, events and experiences to help them connect to their past. By doing this, it gives people some comfort and helps them to retain a better sense of who they are. It is also said to aid memory. Reminiscence therapy is usually carried out with the aid of tangible prompts and reminders such as family photographs and other familiar and items from the past with particular relevance for the person. Music and video prompts are now increasingly used in reminiscence work. Playing someone a favourite song from their past, for example, can prompt happy memories and promote wellbeing. It also helps them reconnect with family members and friends. Reminiscence has much in common with life story work. This is about working with the person and their family to produce a chronicle of their life and their major life events. It is claimed that this can help people with dementia share their stories and enhance their sense of identity. Dementia UK (2017) has produced a template for people wanting to make a life story book – available at www.dementiauk.org/wp-content/uploads/2017/03/Lifestory-.compressed.pdf. This is worth downloading to get a better idea of how life story books are produced and what they can contain.

Various studies indicate that the approaches discussed can be effective but are not necessarily for all people with dementia and not at every point in their lives. There is no conclusive evidence base as yet for the efficacy of any of these approaches. However, much of the anecdotal evidence for reminiscence, life story work and validation therapy suggests that, when used appropriately, these approaches help boost self-esteem and promote wellbeing.

Various elements of all these therapies can be found in dementia care practice today. If anything, they can tend to be used rather eclectically and, because they are predominantly used in care home settings, they are always practised by psychologists or other suitably trained staff. As with so many therapies, what seems to matter most is how they are put into practice rather than the underlying 'theory' behind them.

## Dementia-ism

Dementia-ism is a term coined to describe how people with dementia suffer 'a double jeopardy of age and cognitive disability' (Brooker, 2004: 217). This refers to the idea that deeply embedded discriminatory attitudes still exist in society both towards people in old age and also towards people with diminished cognitive abilities. Therefore, to be in both categories as many people with dementia are negatively affects all aspects of their life. As discussed in Chapter 1, people with dementia not only have to face the disabling impact of the disease, they also have to endure being stereotyped, stigmatised and disempowered through the persistence of negative social attitudes attached to dementia. One of the criticisms of individualised, person-centred approaches, such as Kitwood's, is that they do not take sufficient account of dementia-ism. As Innes (2009) points out, they need to be 'grounded in an understanding of wider structural forces' (p. 19). Improving the lives of people with dementia, therefore, requires work at the personal level but also at the cultural and societal level.

## The VIPS model

The VIPS model is perhaps the most widely known model of person-centred care for people with dementia currently in operation in the UK. It was developed by

Dawn Brooker who was greatly influenced by Tom Kitwood (Brooker, 2007). For example, the model incorporates Kitwood's ideas about malignant social psychology and positive person work. Brooker's aim is to ensure that all those involved in caring for people with dementia are able to understand the principles of person-centred care, identify and overcome any barriers and apply them in practice. To this end, Brooker developed a VIPS Framework© (Brooker, 2007; Brooker and Latham, 2016) so that managers and practitioners could monitor, evidence and reflect on how VIPS principles are put into practice. The development of this framework answers some of the criticisms that have been made about person-centred approaches being too open to interpretation and leaving matters of accountability and, ultimately, enforcement unaddressed. It has also been used as an evaluative tool for researchers (Reilly and Houghton, 2019). Whilst the emphasis of VIPS is on practical application in care settings, Brooker says more than Kitwood did about the need to combat both ageism and, specifically, dementia-ism in wider society.

According to Brooker (2007) VIPS stands for:

**Valuing** people with dementia and those who care for them: promoting citizenship rights and entitlements regardless of age or cognitive impairment, and rooting out discriminatory practice (p. 27).

**Individualised** care. Treating people as individuals: appreciating that people have a unique history and personality, physical and mental health, and social and economic resources, and that these will affect their responses to dementia (p. 44).

**Personal** Perspectives. Looking at the world from the perspective of the person with dementia: recognising that each person's experience has its own validity, that people with dementia act from this perspective, and that empathy with this perspective has its own therapeutic potential (p. 63).

**Social** Environment. Providing a supportive social environment: recognising that all human life is grounded in relationships and that people with dementia need an enriched social environment which both compensates for their impairment and fosters opportunities for personal growth (p. 82).

Evaluations of the VIPS model in practice find that, when applied properly according to the principles, it can promote wellbeing and reduce depression and other neuropsychiatric symptoms in people with dementia. However, one of the biggest challenges to its successful implementation is establishing a culture of care where VIPS principles are fully embedded in organisational practices. It not only needs resources, it requires leadership, training and ongoing monitoring (Røsvik et al., 2011). This highlights that, for a variety of reasons, many care environments do not support the putting into practice of person-centred approaches in the way in which they are intended (Reilly and Houghton, 2019). This can be because of a lack of time, a lack of resources, staff turnover, a lack of support from management, the lack of a dementia trained workforce or all of these. Person-centred approaches also demand a lot of family carers who need proper support in order to maintain their own wellbeing and play an effective role in supporting the person with dementia (Innes, 2009).

## Rights approaches

Unlike writers such as Kitwood and Cheston and Bender, Brooker gives more attention to promoting the 'citizenship rights and entitlements' of people with dementia. As discussed in Chapter 1, the All-Party Parliamentary Group on Dementia (2019) has backed the adoption of a social model of disability and, in doing so, accepted that people with dementia come under the definition of disability provided by the UNCRPD (2006). This does not mean that all people with dementia would necessarily identify themselves as 'disabled', but they would still be protected under the UN Convention and the Equality Act 2010 in the UK nevertheless (Shakespeare, Zeilig and Mittler, 2019). A major factor in the development of social models of disability was people with physical disabilities wanting to push back against the power of health and social professionals to define them and control their lives. They also argued strongly that societies disabled people rather than the impairments they might have. Therefore, disability rights activists demanded that society change to accommodate people with disabilities rather than the other way round (Shakespeare, 2006). In this vein, Gilliard et al. (2005) explain that:

> A social model theory makes us confront the ways in which we discriminate against people with dementia and marginalize all people with dementia in the way services are designed and delivered. It asks uncomfortable questions about whether or not the dementia care 'industry' works to the advantage of people with dementia.
>
> (p. 582)

This raises some difficult questions about the extent to which people with dementia can be not just cared for properly but genuinely empowered within the existing health and social care system. Rights-based approaches go beyond models of 'care' in this respect. To give people rights places duties and obligations on others (either people or organisations) to uphold those rights. It makes them accountable in law. The rights conferred through the Human Rights Act 1998 and Equality Act 2010 not only makes others legally accountable, but it also gives the person legal rights of challenge and, potentially, of redress if it can be shown that their rights have not been upheld. Adopting a rights approach to dementia care gives a more solid legislative framework to person-centred principles and has been endorsed by the World Health Organization (2015b). It also helps promote empowerment and social inclusion by providing formal processes to challenge unfair treatment and combat discrimination. Case Study 4.1 is based on an example provided by the World Health Organization (2015b: 4).

## Case Study 4.1:   Charter on human rights and people living with dementia, Scotland, United Kingdom

In Scotland, it was recognised that people living with dementia are entitled to the same human rights as everyone else. Nevertheless, people living with dementia were still often being denied their rights due to social and cultural barriers. These barriers included a lack of understanding within the population and a lack of training for care staff in how to respect and protect the human rights of people living with dementia. Therefore, in 2009, the Scottish parliament adopted the human rights-based approach to dementia, 'PANEL'. The aim was to uphold the human rights of people living with dementia both in the community and in care facilities in Scotland.

PANEL stands for:

**P** Participation – Everyone has the right to participate in decisions that affect them. Participation must be active, free, meaningful and give attention to issues of accessibility, including access to information in a form and a language that can be understood.
**A** Accountability – Requires effective monitoring of human rights standards as well as effective remedies for human rights breaches.
**N** Non-discrimination and equality – A human rights-based approach means that all forms of discrimination in the realisation of rights must be prohibited, prevented and eliminated.
**E** Empowerment – Individuals and communities should understand their rights and should be fully supported to participate in the development of policy and practices which affect their lives.
**L** Legality – A human rights-based approach requires the recognition of rights as legally enforceable entitlements and is linked to national and international human rights law.

The PANEL framework fleshes out what was discussed earlier about rights-based approaches establishing lines of accountability and introducing enforceability in law. However, as it also makes clear, people must be supported to know, understand and utilise their rights when necessary. Being able to participate in decisions and to understand and utilise rights becomes difficult, if not impossible, as dementia progresses for many people. Therefore, the embedding of rights into

person-centred approaches does not remove the typical dilemmas associated with caring for people with dementia, such as how to safeguard
and best support people assessed to be vulnerable without compro-
mising their rights to choice, privacy and self-determination. How is it
decided, for example, what is in someone's best interests if they lack
the capacity to make that decision themselves? These questions come
down to professional judgement, the application of values and careful
application of principles set out in codes of practice.

For practitioners in the UK and England, the following publications
are recommended:

*Dementia and Human Rights: A practitioner's guide.* British Institute of
Human Rights (2016a).
*Social Care Intervention and Human Rights: A practitioner's guide.* British
Institute of Human Rights (2016b).
*Supporting people living with dementia to be involved in adult safe-
guarding enquiries* (Department of Health and Social Care, 2021).

## Palliative care

The *Prime Minister's challenge on dementia 2020* (Department of Health, 2015a)
talked about 'all people with dementia and their carers' having access to high-
quality palliative care from health and social care staff trained in dementia. Palliative care is defined as 'the active holistic care of people with advanced, progressive
illness' (NICE, 2021). It is about maintaining someone's quality of life if they have
a life-limiting condition, making sure, for example, that pain is managed properly
and that they end their life with dignity and in as much comfort as possible. It is
also about making sure that the person's caregivers are supported. Palliative care is
not just for people in their very last days of life, it can be offered to anyone with
an incurable condition that will shorten their life. Palliative care can therefore be
offered to someone for weeks or months, even years. Palliative care can be provided
in someone's own home, in a specialist setting such as a hospice or another care setting such as a care home. It is usually provided by a multi-disciplinary team which
can include doctors, nurses, social workers and different types of therapists.

Palliative care is not a specific model of dementia care. However, because
dementia is recognised as a terminal illness (SCIE, 2020), thinking about palliative
care becomes more relevant as the disease progresses, the person becomes less and
less able to look after themselves and needs more nursing and medical attention as
they approach their death. People in the advanced stages of dementia can become
dehydrated or suffer serious weight loss because of losing the ability to chew and

swallow (oral motor skills) and because they might not be able to recognise that they are hungry and thirsty. They also have a greater chance of catching infections and are less able to cope with the effects of other illnesses and ongoing conditions (de Vries, 2003; Froggatt and Goodman, 2014). They might become depressed, experience anxiety and have difficulty with sleeping or just getting comfortable. Cognitive and communication problems can make it harder to determine how the person is feeling and whether they are in any pain or discomfort. Having dementia does not mean that it is always the cause of someone's death, people with dementia more often die from a combination of factors. Therefore, a person might not die 'from' dementia but their dementia might well have been a contributory factor in their death. The thought of palliative care can raise some difficult emotional and practical issues for the person and their caregivers, not least because it involves thinking and talking about death and dying. Many health and social care professionals also do not find such conversations easy to have (Department of Health, 2008).

There are questions to consider not only about *how* to have conversations about end-of-life matters but also *when*. The current advice recommends that early conversations with people with dementia are important so that people can plan ahead for their future care, including palliative and end-of-life care (Alzheimer's Society, 2021d). However, the question is what constitutes 'early'? Froggatt and Goodman (2014) ask whether it is 'appropriate to be raising issues of mortality and dying when a person is only just coming to terms with a diagnosis?' (p. 367). Possibly 'timely' is a more appropriate way of looking at it. Some people never come to terms with their diagnosis, but even for those who do, decisions about how to prepare for one's end of life and when to start the conversation are always likely to be difficult. Another complicating factor is that it can be difficult to predict exactly when someone with dementia is nearing death. They might present with signs that suggest they are very close to death, but they might continue in that state for many months or even years. They may seem near to death and then improve and live for many months longer (SCIE, 2020).

For some, end-of-life care might raise questions about the possibility of assisted dying. This subject has many legal, ethical as well as clinical implications (Tomlinson and Stott, 2015). Assisted dying (euthanasia) is currently illegal in the UK and many other countries, but is, nevertheless, a matter of ongoing debate internationally (Jakhar, Ambreen and Prasad, 2021). There is always the possibility that the topic might arise in the context of planning end-of-life care, but it is not a matter that social workers have a professional mandate or responsibility to advise on. However, people who want to discuss these issues can be directed to the NHS website www.nhs.uk/conditions/euthanasia-and-assisted-suicide/ or websites such as that of Dignity In Dying (www.dignityindying.org.uk/your-rights/) which clarify the legal position in the UK.

These issues and challenges notwithstanding, health and social care professionals should be prepared to intervene at the earliest possible stage and have the necessary conversations with people with dementia and their caregivers. Unfortunately, the

Care Quality Commission (2016) reported that people with dementia in England experience poorer quality care at the end of their lives than others because providers and commissioners do not always understand or fully consider their specific needs. Among the barriers that prevent people with dementia from receiving good end-of-life care are: lack of identification and planning, unequal access to care, and poor quality of care (Care Quality Commission, 2016). This paints quite a grim picture but underlines the need for health and social care professionals to be prepared not just to have conversations with people with dementia and their carers about end-of-life care but also to advocate for better services within the health and social care system.

## Advanced Care Planning

Dementia is a progressive disease that impacts on people's ability to make informed decisions about important matters in their life. For people with dementia ACP is, therefore, an important element to palliative care. It offers the opportunity to plan future care and support, including medical treatment, whilst the person still has the mental capacity to do so. The *Prime Minister's challenge on dementia 2020* (Department of Health, 2015a) states that all people with a diagnosis of dementia should be given the opportunity for ACP early in the course of their illness, including plans for the end of life. Although it can be difficult to face death and the challenges it brings, people with dementia communicating their care and treatment preferences in advance, allows everyone involved to prepare for any future eventualities as best as possible. ACP can help relieve some of the burdens of responsibility on family caregivers having to make decisions when they might not necessarily know (or care in some cases) about what the person considers to be in their best interests. ACP cannot take all the stress out of end-of-life care decisions but it can mitigate it. However, as the following extract indicates, it does involve people grasping the nettle and being frank with each other:

---

**BOX 4.1 TINA WORMLEY, EXPERT BY EXPERIENCE IN 'MY FUTURE WISHES' (NHS ENGLAND, 2018: 6)**

If we are to offer ACPs to people with dementia, then we need to be frank with them. Dementia is a terminal disease; you don't recover from it. We do not avoid this language with other terminal diseases. It puts patients with dementia at a serious disadvantage. It strips them of their right to make choices about their care. It has to be done early before loss of capacity occurs. Two years into the disease and my mum could not have truly understood the implications of an ACP. At the very beginning, she could have.

---

## Advance decisions and advance statements

People thinking about the impact their dementia might have on their mental capacity and, therefore, their ability to make decisions about their care and support as their health deteriorates, can make advance decisions and advance statements. An advance decision can be a written or spoken statement that sets out refusals of treatment. It is legally binding as long as the relevant procedures in the Mental Capacity Act 2005 are followed. If the person wants to refuse life-sustaining treatment, they must put this in writing, sign and date it in the presence of a witness who also must sign and date it. If a certain type of medical treatment is asked for, as opposed to refusing one, it should be taken into account but it will not legally bind a doctor or professional to follow it. To be valid, the person must have mental capacity at the time it was made. If the person sets up a LPA for health and care decisions which gives an attorney the power to make decisions about treatments, doctors are free to follow the LPA's directions rather than those in the advance decision.

An advance statement is a statement of someone's general wishes and care preferences. For example, where they would like to live, or the type of care and support they want to receive. It is not legally binding, although it should be referred to when decisions are being made in best interests decisions.

ACP and thinking ahead about end-of-life decisions are important considerations in palliative care. However, in a study focusing on ACP in dementia care, Robinson et al. (2013) found there was a lack of clarity about which professionals should be responsible for ACP. This meant that there were delays in initiating ACP and opportunities for planning were not provided whilst the patient still had capacity. Perhaps more alarming they conclude:

> Our data reveal that professionals exhibit considerable reserve about the value of ACP; this is in contrast to national policy initiatives promoting it. Despite the practical issues they encounter, this appears to be fundamentally related to a belief that their care systems are not adequate to meet patient wishes, especially in dementia care. It may, however, be due to a degree of pragmatic fatalism that one can never plan ahead for all the possible future scenarios. This mirrors the findings of research exploring older peoples, including those living with dementia, views on ACP. They are reluctant to engage in ACP adopting a 'hoping for the best' attitude and prefer to trust their family or family physician to take responsibility for health-care decisions, although relatives of people with dementia find proxy decision-making very difficult, especially at the end of life.
> *(Robinson et al., 2013: 406)*

This aspect of palliative care is clearly an area where more clarity and more resource is needed. However, on one level, it is easy to see how many people, including professionals, might adopt a 'hoping for the best' attitude. Death, dying and planning for the end of life are difficult subjects. However, in order to ensure good care and support for people with dementia in the latter stages of the disease, practitioners must be prepared to both facilitate and engage in communication in this area. For one reason, it might avoid some of the feelings of regret, failure and guilt that can emerge among carers when such conversations are avoided (Harrop et al., 2016).

## Concluding comments

This chapter has discussed selected approaches to supporting and caring for people with dementia, including palliative and end-of-life care. It has discussed how the bio-medical model has been challenged by approaches that are more 'person-centred' and rights-based. However, the bio-medical model remains strong due, amongst other things, to the power of the medical profession and the desire to find a cure and better treatments for dementia through bio-medical science. It has been argued that rights-based approaches make service commissioners and providers more accountable and should help in promoting empowerment and social inclusion as well as a good standard of person-centred care for people with dementia. An ongoing challenge is to combat dementia-ism.

Although they take place in a multi-disciplinary context, much of the impetus for these approaches has come from the nursing profession. Nursing and other health care staff also undertake much of the direct work with people with dementia, particularly as the disease progresses. Whilst it might not be as 'hands-on' as some professions that work with people with dementia, social work has an important part to play. It is, therefore, essential to understand the principles that underpin and the concepts that inform contemporary approaches to dementia care. Chapter 5 focuses more specifically on the social work role and discusses how social workers can play a full part in promoting good dementia care as part of a multi-disciplinary response.

## Further reading

Kitwood, T. and Brooker, D. (Eds). (2019). *Dementia Reconsidered, Revisited: The Person Still Comes First*. London: Open University Press.

As discussed, Tom Kitwood made an important contribution towards introducing a 'new' culture of person-centred dementia care. This book includes the substance of Kitwood's original book. However, the editor, Dawn Brooker, has drawn together different commentaries which revisit and update it, including many of the points raised in this chapter.

Brooker, D. (2007). *Person-Centred Dementia Care. Making Services Better*. London: Jessica Kingsley Publishers.

Brooker, D. and Latham, I. (2016). *Person-Centred Dementia Care. Making Services Better with the VIPS Framework* (2nd edition). London: Jessica Kingsley Publishers.

Dawn Brooker is a major figure in dementia studies in the UK and continues to research and teach about different aspects of dementia care. The publications listed set out both the background to and the principles of her VIPS model. The emphasis is on how VIPS principles should be put into practice.

# 5

# THE SOCIAL WORK ROLE

## Knowledge, skills and values

By the end of this chapter, you should have an understanding of:

- Why and how social workers become involved with people living with dementia and their carers.
- The social work role with people living with dementia in different settings.
- The social work skills, knowledge and values required in order to work effectively with people living with dementia and their carers.

## Setting the scene

Earlier chapters explained that dementia is a complex phenomenon where neither the experiences nor the needs of individual people living with it cannot be taken for granted. It was also explained that, despite this being the case, people with dementia are still stereotyped, pigeonholed and discriminated against in society. Chapter 2 set out the broader contexts in which social work with people takes place. Current policy requires dementia services to be person-centred, rights-based, non-discriminatory and inclusive. However, it was noted that whilst the importance of providing good dementia care and support has been established in policy agendas in recent years, the health and social care system in the UK, of which social work is part, has come under increasing strain for different reasons. Chapter 4 explained that, whilst social work has an integral role to play as part of a multi-disciplinary response to supporting people with dementia, it differs in some important respects from the nursing and caring role, where contact with the person with dementia can be more intimate and take place over longer periods of time. This is, to some extent, a generalisation; however, the exact nature of the social work role will vary depending on the specific context and setting in which it takes place. Therefore, social work practices with people with dementia need to be situated in their various contexts for the discussion

DOI: 10.4324/9781003191667-6

to fully make sense. Much of the broader social, economic, legislative and policy contexts have been covered in previous chapters. However, social work always takes place in an organisational context and in a particular practice climate or environment. It is important to understand the characteristics and demands of these more ground-level contexts in order to practise professionally and prepare effectively for and meet the challenges associated with them. It is not really helpful to talk about social work out of context. The challenge is to practise professionally within the constraints that exist in the real world.

## Settings

Social work with people with dementia takes place in the community (usually the person's own home); care homes; hospitals of different kinds and other care settings such as hospices. The same person might receive services in different settings at different times. In the UK, local authorities can organise their services differently. However, most of the work undertaken with people with dementia is undertaken by community-based adult social work teams. Many areas also operate more specialist, multi-disciplinary older people's mental health teams. Often there can be disputes about whether a person becomes the responsibility of one team or another. A medical diagnosis usually decides, but that is not always the case. Different teams can have their own local eligibility criteria and agreements. Hospital social work teams usually take responsibility when the person has been admitted to hospital and is awaiting discharge. Again, there can be some 'territorial' tensions around issues, such as when someone known to a community team is admitted to hospital and then discharged. In cases when the person is not already known to a community team, there can be disagreements about who takes responsibility for the person and at what point. This can lead to delays in receiving help. The community-hospital social work interface is a test of collaborative working and needs to be managed well or else the person can either slip through the net; they and their carers can be confused about who is looking after them and there can be delays in services (Holder et al., 2018). Changes in living arrangements especially hospital admission can trigger distress, confusion and delirium for someone with dementia. Therefore when people with dementia move from one setting to another, it is absolutely vital for them and their carers that the service is seamless and that any changes are explained clearly and in a timely fashion. For this to happen successfully, the professionals involved must also communicate with each other in a clear and timely fashion, and keep the service user and carers in the loop at all times.

## Tasks

The broad aims of adult social work are helping people to live independently as much as possible; promoting wellbeing and safeguarding people who are vulnerable from the risk of harm (BASW, 2018). With these broad aims in mind, the main tasks of social work with people with dementia include: carrying out assessments (e.g. of need, risk, mental capacity and of carers' needs); planning personalised care and support; arranging, monitoring and reviewing care and support; safeguarding; making referrals and signposting to other services and advocacy. Hospital-based social work is usually closely connected to discharge planning. The role of social workers in palliative care settings means that, in addition to the tasks mentioned earlier, they become more involved in counselling and bereavement support (Association of Palliative Care Social Workers, 2016).

## Triggers for social work involvement

There are several sets of circumstances in which social workers come into contact with people living with dementia and their carers. These include:

- Concerns expressed by family members, neighbours or professionals such as GPs or District Nurses about the person's physical and mental health deteriorating to the point that they are unable to cope on their own, live independently and without risk of harm.
- Carer stress and carers who are no longer able to cope in the role. The primary carers for many older people with dementia are their spouses, who might also have physical and mental impairments of their own. Referrals can be made by the carer themselves or by others concerned about their wellbeing.
- Referrals from sheltered housing schemes and care homes because the person's health has deteriorated and they need extra care or the referrer thinks that the person needs to be moved to a more appropriate setting.
- A crisis. For example, the death or illness of the main carer. It could also be an unexpected health incident or accident experienced by the person themselves such as a fall.
- Safeguarding concerns. It is suspected that either the person is at risk of harm from someone, is actually experiencing some kind of abuse or that they might be seriously self-neglecting.

The list is not exhaustive but covers many of the main reasons why social workers become involved with people living with dementia. Sometimes there is plenty of time to gather information and plan but in other circumstances, action needs to be taken urgently. It is important that the principles of seeking the person's views and respecting their rights need to be followed whatever the circumstances.

## Framing

Social workers need to be attentive to how referrals for social work are framed or worded. We should ask ourselves how the person and their situation are being constructed. Referrals can often (unconsciously) reflect the stereotyped ways of thinking and speaking about dementia discussed in Chapter 1. The language used to frame referrals and inform other communication regarding a person with dementia can imply certain preferred courses of action, whilst ruling out others. Again, this can militate against using a person–centred approach if a label is applied to someone even before the first contact has been made.

---

**BOX 5.1   ACTIVITY 5.1**

The mobile warden responsible for a sheltered housing scheme gets in touch to request social work intervention with Maud who lives in one of the sheltered flats under her supervision. She says 'We think the world of poor old Maudie, but we all think that her dementia is getting to the point that she's going to have to move. She's wandering, bothering other residents and generally making a nuisance of herself. Also, she was spotted out in the middle of the road the other night, just in her nightie. She's not safe. We'll be sorry to see her go but I think she's needs something more 24/7. It's only going to get worse. She could end up doing herself a lot of harm at this rate. Also, it's not fair on the others'.

**To think about**

What are your thoughts about the way this referral has been made and Maud constructed? Do you think that we have a balanced view of Maud, the person, and her world? How might you ensure that Maud receives a response that is person-centred, rights-based, non-discriminatory and inclusive?

---

Many of the issues raised in this activity will be covered later in the chapter. However, it should be noted that it is not uncommon, even amongst professionals, to take a fatalistic and deterministic approach to living with dementia. Referrers can also stress specific aspects of someone's behaviour or situation to create urgency and to guide other agencies to take their preferred course of action – often without the person's knowledge or consent. Therefore, it is important that the process in which someone becomes a 'referral' and then constituted as a 'case' in the social work system is examined critically for inappropriate or stereotyped labels and other forms of dementia-ism.

## Challenges in the practice environment

Unfortunately, that is not the only challenge facing social workers in their practice with people living with dementia. As discussed in Chapter 2, adult social work and social care are stretched in many ways. Whilst there are local variations, in overall terms, there are not enough social workers, caseloads are high and there is a lack of resources, including time to do the job properly (Ravalier and Boichat, 2018). As a consequence, providing satisfactory outcomes for service users is far from guaranteed (Moriarty and Manthorpe, 2016). Hospital social workers have their own specific issues. The nature of the work is fast-paced and they often have limited contact with the people with whom they work. This can involve having just one contact with the person concerned (Gibbons and Plath, 2006). Hospital social workers report that heavy caseloads are the biggest barrier they face in providing support to people in hospital at the end of their lives (McCormick et al., 2007). On a more positive note, Moriarty and Manthorpe (2016) found that, whilst there is evidence of unmet demand, there is considerable satisfaction with palliative care social workers among service users and carers. This could reflect that social workers in these settings have better opportunities to form relationships with service users.

Practising social work with people with dementia is a complex task requiring a high level of skill and knowledge. The main reason for setting the scene in this way is to make the point that, in order to practise effectively, social workers need to meet certain challenges and be able to surmount several obstacles. For example, characteristics of the wider system and the organisational context in which social work takes place can mean that important tasks need to be undertaken on limited time and, sometimes, in suboptimal conditions. Despite this, it is important not to lose sight of the basic principles of social work and of good dementia care. Also, whilst the pressure can be to deal with immediate practical problems, combatting discriminatory attitudes towards people living with dementia should be regarded as an important ongoing task.

## Social work skills

The core skills that social workers need to possess, at all levels, and in any setting, are laid out in the Professional Capabilities Framework (PCF), specifically in Domain Seven (BASW, 2018). Given the particular challenges of practising social work with people with dementia that have been highlighted, the main focus here will be on the skills of communication, empathy, forming relationships, assessment and advocacy. However, it should be noted that these need to be underpinned by other important social work skills such as reflective practice and multi-disciplinary working.

### *Communication*

Effective communication skills are an essential component of social work. Through different types of communication we give and gather information, express empathy, build relationships and carry out assessments (Lishman, 2009; Henderson and Mathew-Byrne, 2016). However, as discussed in Chapter 2, different types of dementia can make communication more difficult. This might be through difficulties with speech, vision, hearing, facial expressions and memory as well as other cognitive impairments. A person's ability to communicate depends on several factors, including what type of dementia they have and what stage in the disease they are at. Broader cultural and social factors such as the person's ethnicity and social class also come into play, although it is important not to make assumptions about these (Botsford and Harrison Dening, 2015). Therefore, person-centred social work interventions require the social worker to avoid making generalisations based on labels and to adapt their communication to the particular needs and situation of the person.

In managing successful communication with people with dementia, it is useful to refer back to Kitwood's concepts of malign social psychology and positive person work. Kitwood (1997) made the point that the quality of communication between people contributes towards how they feel about themselves as human beings. Consequently, social workers need to pay close attention to the interrelationship of a set of factors that can impact on communication.

## Empathy: tuning in to self and others

Empathy is the ability to try to imagine what is like to be the other person in order to understand their feelings. It is also the ability to communicate this understanding back to them (Lishman, 2009). Kadushin and Kadushin (2013) argue that the skill of 'anticipatory empathy' helps us to understand any concerns or anxieties that someone might have about us or the situation that they are in. Anticipatory empathy also helps correct the tendency to stereotype other people based on generalised knowledge. However, Killick and Allan (2001) acknowledge that if we do not have direct experience of living with dementia this is difficult. Nevertheless, they proposed that with imagination and experience it should be possible to some extent. It is never something that can be taken for granted though. Empathising with people with dementia is not necessarily straightforward but is something that needs to be worked at and practised. SCIE and organisations such as the Alzheimer's Society have produced videos that aim to convey something of what it is like to live dementia. *Dementia from the inside* (SCIE, 2015) is a good example www.youtube.com/watch?v=Erjzl1WL8yQ. These videos are useful but obviously cannot capture the particular, subjective experiences of a specific individual.

Kitwood (1997) talks about the importance of 'I Thou' relationship and the importance of remembering the person behind the dementia. Using their chosen name as often as appropriate is helpful in establishing such a relationship. It has a symbolic function as it helps preserve their individuality and dignity and it has a practical function because it helps the person concentrate on what is being said.

An equally useful concept to help underpin communication with people with dementia is that of 'tuning in', as developed by Shulman (2008). Basically, this means that before and during interactions with service users, social workers should use critical reflection to get in touch with (tune into) their own feelings about the meeting. This can help with identifying unhelpful prejudices or preconceptions or any other pre-existing concerns that might influence the outcome. For example, is anything being projected onto the person because of a particular medical label or because of something written or spoken in a referral? Social workers should also aim to 'tune into' the world of the person they are meeting in order to try and pick up what they are feeling and gain a sense of their inner world. For example, what feelings, anxieties or concerns might they be bringing to their interaction with you? Managing effective communication in social work requires emotional intelligence (Morrison, 2006). Apart from being aware of any emotional baggage they might be carrying, social workers need to be able to read the emotional climate, get a sense of any anxiety, irritation or confusion in the other person, understand why it might be there and manage it sensitively.

## Physical environment

Attending to the physical environment in which communication takes place is as important as attending to the emotional environment. It is essential to find a quiet, private, calm space with no distractions (Killick and Allan, 2001; Department of Health, 2015b). This would be true for most social work conversations, but the cognitive and other issues associated with dementia mean that the person needs every assistance in understanding what is being said and in being as fully engaged with what is going on as possible. Social workers who assess people in hospitals can have a particularly challenging task in finding a suitable environment. Some anticipatory and preparatory work with ward staff is useful in this respect. Even if you think you have found the perfect location, the person should be asked if it suits them. This also has a symbolic value. It conveys that the person has a choice about where they discuss their personal matters.

## Tone

The tone of spoken communication with people with dementia needs to be warm, engaging, respectful and reassuring but without infantilizing or patronizing the person in the process. Tone is conveyed through voice and the choice of language and through non-verbal communication such as facial expression and other gestures. Throughout meetings, our tone needs to be continually monitored and checked in line with the other person's reactions to ensure that we have not strayed into either being too formal, too informal or patronising. This is an ongoing process of reflexive fine-tuning, especially when meeting someone for the first time.

## Non-verbal communication

Attention to non-verbal communication is especially important as many people living with dementia have a heightened awareness of others' body language (Killick and Allan, 2001). Non-verbal communication, therefore, needs to be congruent with verbal communication in establishing tone. This means maintaining appropriate eye contact and conveying attentiveness through our facial expression, posture and other gestures (for example, orientating ourselves to the person). The overall tone of our verbal and non-verbal communication needs to convey that we are interested in that person and that we are taking them seriously.

For many people with dementia, as the disease progresses, memory deteriorates and word retrieval becomes more difficult. Non-verbal communication becomes an increasingly important way of expressing their feelings and needs (Allen, 2001; Parker, 2003). Social workers need to be sensitive to non-verbal communication and avoid jumping to conclusions. For example, people who have been living with the disease for some time can develop facial expressions that are expressionless or they might wear an almost permanent frown. These facial expressions might not necessarily reflect their inner world. The important thing is not to take this as disapproval, rejection or lack of interest, but to keep engaged and to keep going unless the person makes it very obvious that they do not want to talk to you. Facial expression alone is often not enough. It needs to be read in conjunction with other non-verbal communication such as gestures and non-verbal vocalisations. Non-verbal vocalisations such as groaning or screaming can become more apparent as the disease progresses. It is important that these are not dismissed as meaningless signs of agitation. Non-verbal vocalisations can present strong clues to how the person is feeling and what they want to communicate (Hyden, 2011). Whilst carers can be asked for their interpretations, social workers should be prepared to keep an open mind, at least until they get to know the person better.

Because different types of dementia present different communication problems at different stages, the use of pictograms, photographs and other symbols has proved useful to overcome problems with verbal communication (Allen, 2001; Parker, 2003; Banovic, Zunic and Sinanovic, 2018). However, unless confident and trained in these methods of communication, social workers should be cautious about using them without checking with people who know the person, in case the method causes more confusion. However, it is an option to consider and is used effectively in care settings, for example, to establish preferences over meals and so on. It is a useful tool to have in one's repertoire once sufficient homework has been done on what works best for that particular person.

### Proxemics

Proxemics is a sub-category of non-verbal communication which refers to how interpersonal space is used (Lishman, 2009). Establishing the appropriate physical distance is important. Too close can be intimidating, too far might create a barrier and suggest remoteness and lack of interest. Judgment about proxemics also needs to take into account any visual or hearing impairments, which are increasingly common as the disease progresses. As a rule of thumb, it is useful to have one's head on the same level as the person to whom you are talking, so they do not have to look up or down to see your face and facial expressions. Attending to proxemics has a symbolic function as well as a practical one because it lets the person know that you are focusing on them whilst respecting their boundaries. There are also social and cultural dimensions to proxemics to take into account. This might apply to certain ethnic or religious groups and in relation to gender differences. Rather than make some generalised prescriptions about these, the most appropriate course of action is, first, to be aware of the importance of proxemics and, second, to take cues from the person and take advice from those who know them well as to what is appropriate.

## Timing and pace

Attention to the timing and pace of discussions with people with dementia is particularly important in order to avoid, inadvertently, 'outpacing' them. This is the term that Kitwood (1997) used to describe the process whereby information and choices are presented at a rate too fast for the person to understand. This is more likely to happen when time is short and work schedules are busy but must be resisted if malignant social psychology is to be avoided (Killick and Allan, 2001). Therefore, when meeting, it is useful to allow time at the start for the person to orientate themselves to you and to clarify with them what they understand the purpose of your meeting is. It is not uncommon for people with dementia, aware of their cognitive deficits, to want to 'perform' well socially. This means that effort goes into concealing communication problems and making it seem as if levels of comprehension are better than they are. So, it is important not to take anything for granted and check the person's understanding regularly and make sure that the pace of the meeting is comfortable for the person. Checking is useful because it can provide valuable clues about the person's level of comprehension as well as their memory.

Empathetic 'tuning in' to the other person is required to ensure that the pace does not slow to the point of being patronising for that individual. Person-centredness involves constant fine-tuning of all aspects of our communication.

## Clarity

Another communication technique to facilitate comprehension is to keep sentences short and limited to one point at a time. So, for example, in everyday discourse we might say:

> *Given what you now know about your diagnosis and how it is affecting you, what do you think is the best way forward for you, for example, is it something that particularly worries you, what are the things that most bother you? Memory maybe? Leaving the gas on? What sort of things have you talked over with your wife. Money? Getting out and about? Shopping? That kind of thing really. It could be anything. I suppose there are long term concerns and more pressing short term ones. So what sort of things are you worried about managing?*

Even though, as a social worker, you might want to touch on these topics, that is far too long and rambling. It contains multiple questions and jumps from topic to topic. It asks about their feelings, different practical issues, discussions with the wife, long- and short-term concerns. If it had a thread, it would be hard to follow it and make a coherent response. It would be simpler for the person if the conversation started with an opening question such as 'How do you think your illness is affecting you?' and then, having allowed the person to answer that in their own words, ask them about the other points, one at a time, preferably in ways that follow on logically from what they have said. To achieve clarity, it is important to avoid jargon and think about which forms of words are most likely to be understood by that person (Allen, 2001). Frequent checking back and the use of paraphrasing are important in order to ensure as much clarity in the communication as possible (Lishman, 2009).

## Listening and observation

Active listening is an essential component in all social work communication (Lishman, 2009; Trevithick, 2012). However, the need to stay silent, listen and observe is particularly important in communication with people with dementia. This allows them, amongst other things, to absorb what is going on, think, retrieve words and formulate the response they want to make (Killick and Allan, 2001). So, sometimes a brake needs to be put on how active the listening is – not too many encouraging nods for example. This can apply unnecessary pressure. In fact, it is probably more appropriate to think in terms of 'empathetic listening'. This involves paying particular attention to the emotional themes and messages that lie beneath what is being said and reacting accordingly. It is not uncommon for people living with dementia to say things that you know to be factually untrue, such as a 93-year-old woman saying that they are waiting for their mother to come home from work. This statement does not need to be challenged or endorsed. The empathetic listener acknowledges that they have heard what the person has said and conveys to them that this is something that has meaning for them. Whilst it most likely indicates that the person is expressing a longing for emotional security or comfort, it is not really that helpful to share this interpretation with them either. The important thing is just to recognise it. The next section discusses possible responses when you are aware that there is no factual basis to what someone with dementia is saying.

Attentive, empathetic listening, whilst paying attention to non-verbal communication, is at the heart of good communication practice with people with dementia. However, it can require a degree of silence that might be unusual in other social work situations.

Observation is an important skill in all social work practice (O'Loughlin and O'Loughlin, 2015), but particularly useful in social work with dementia (Department of Health, 2015b). Most observation in social work is unlikely to be anything like as structured as that used in DCM. Social workers usually do not have the time, even if they wanted to undertake this particular kind of observation. It will usually take place naturally, whilst meeting with someone for assessment or some other purpose. Observation is more useful if it has a focus. So, for example, if someone is considered to be at risk in the kitchen, it is useful to observe the person in that particular context. It can be suggested that you might want to accompany them to the kitchen to make a cup of tea. That way it is possible to gain a better sense of the environment in which the person lives and also how they behave in that particular environment. Depending on how capable they are, either they can make the tea, a carer can or, with their permission, the social worker can. The important thing is to observe the person in the appropriate context. Observation is also quite useful in testing and challenging labels that have been applied to people. A carer or relative might talk about an individual's 'challenging' behaviour for example. This can be better understood and put into context better by observing the person's interactions in the environment where they are said to present the behaviour regarded as challenging. Stokes (2000) makes a good point that sometimes people like carers and relatives can be too familiar with someone, to the point that they cease noticing how they actually behave because of preconceptions they might hold about them. A social worker might have limited time, but they come with fresh eyes, they are free from preconceptions and can notice details that others might miss.

### Responding to factual inaccuracies

As indicated earlier, conversations with people with dementia can, at times, lead to situations where the person says something that you are certain is factually inaccurate. This can present a professional dilemma in how to respond. The BASW Code of Ethics for Social Work (2021) is clear that:

> Being trustworthy. Social workers should work in a way that is honest, reliable and open. They should clearly explain their roles, interventions and decisions. They should not seek to deceive or manipulate people who use their services.
>
> *(p. 8)*

Therefore, the fundamental principle is to be honest and not deceitful. However, to correct or challenge certain factually incorrect statements can cause unnecessary distress. Collusion is not necessarily helpful either. Much of the time, it is helpful just to let such statements pass and reflect upon why the person might have said what they did. Nevertheless, it is a difficult area of practice and professional judgement needs to be exercised based on each specific situation. For example, if you arrive for an appointment on a Tuesday and the person is not ready for you because they think it is Monday, it is appropriate to sensitively orientate them to what the day is. However, to engage in lengthy confrontations about other factual inaccuracies such as when someone says they need to go to work (when they retired ten years ago), is not worth pursuing. It is better to try to read what that statement might represent for them. It could mean, for example, a reluctance to engage with you for some reason. For more on this topic, see the section on psychological therapies in Chapter 4 which, for example, discusses the merits of RO versus validation.

Organisations such as the Alzheimer's Society offer very good advice to carers and families on this topic, for example, www.alzheimers.org.uk/get-support/daily-living/making-decisions-telling-truth. They list the following points for carers to consider around telling the truth:

- Is there a message behind the question that indicates an emotion or unmet need, for example, fear, loneliness or disorientation?
- Is the person likely to understand what they are being told? Are there ways of making it easier for them to understand?

- Would knowing the truth cause the person significant distress? If so, would the consequences of telling the truth outweigh the need?
- Are there ways of telling the person the truth that would be less upsetting?
- Are there some things that are essential to be honest about?
- Will not telling the truth make things more difficult in the long run?
- From your knowledge of the person, what do you think they would want?

One of the main reasons for taking a person-centred approach is to tailor responses to what meets the needs of that particular person. Therefore, there is no general formulation to be prescribed. However, with the *Code of Ethics* in mind, social workers should always think seriously about why *not* telling the truth or being honest on a particular occasion is in the person's best interests. The points listed provide a useful checklist in this respect.

## Interpreters

With the population becoming more ethnically diverse, the chances are that social workers will encounter more people with dementia who do not speak English or do not have English as their first language. This complicates communication. The aforementioned points apply in respect of tone, pacing, proxemics and so on are made more challenging when a third party is involved. Although convenient and often the choice of the person, Botsford (2015) cautions against using relatives because it cannot be guaranteed that the messages conveyed will be delivered accurately – both ways. Relatives can be well meaning but have their own agenda. This means that properly trained and approved interpreters need to be used. In such cases, care needs to be taken not to exclude the person by having lengthy conversations with the interpreter. Maintaining a person-centred focus becomes harder. The guidance *Spoken Language Interpreters in Social Work* (Lucas, 2020) is a useful, evidence-based reference in this respect.

## The role of other people

Discussion about interpreters serves as a reminder that often social workers meet people with dementia who are accompanied by other people – most commonly family members or other carers. These people can help facilitate communication and be valuable sources of information because they have pre-existing relationships with that person. However, there are also communication dangers about which to be cautious. Depending on how well the person with dementia can communicate for themselves, the person with them can easily become the person given all the attention, marginalising the person with dementia in the process. In the worst cases, the person with dementia becomes reduced to being talked about as if they were not present. They become a non-person. To avoid this happening, important information from relatives and carers can be exchanged in a separate meeting if necessary. If the person with dementia is physically present in the meeting, every effort has to be made to keep them included, to maintain appropriate levels of eye contact and not to talk over them. A more delicate matter is how to manage any disrespectful language or behaviour shown by the other person at the time. For example, if a wife looks at her husband and says 'Unfortunately, he is just a useless vegetable now'. Rather than challenge this or simply agree, an appropriate response might be to say 'It must be difficult when their dementia means that someone you know well becomes harder to recognise as the person they used to be'. This is neither condemning nor endorsing the comment but acknowledges the person's feelings and the situation they are in, without chastising them in the process. That said, if a repeated pattern of verbally abusive behaviour is observed, this might indicate the need to enact safeguarding procedures. Again, it is a matter of professional judgement based on what has been observed and any other relevant information that can be gathered.

## Assessments and assessment skills

### General overview

Assessments of various kinds are at the heart of social work practice (Coulshed and Orme, 2012; Gaylard, 2013). Carrying out an assessment can sometimes be the only contribution a social worker makes to a particular person's case (Hood, 2016). Therefore, it can be seen as an intervention in its own right. This is an important point because it underlines that the fact of having a social work assessment alone will impact on someone's life in some way. It might be a positive experience, a negative one or both, but it will not be a neutral experience. Therefore, social workers need to think about how the experience of being assessed will leave the person feeling. Will they, for example, feel better about their situation or worse as a consequence? How has the assessment and the way it has been conducted contributed to those feelings? Amongst other considerations, it highlights the importance of taking a strengths-based approach to assessment in adult social work and particularly when working with people with dementia (HM Government, 2014; McGovern, 2015). For many people, having got to a point in their lives where they need to be assessed by a social worker does not make them feel good about themselves. Some argue that being the subject of an assessment can actually be an oppressive experience because of the power imbalance (Coulshed and Orme, 2012). However, the way in which the assessment is conducted can not only mitigate any negative feelings but also leave the person feeling more hopeful. Although they can be a one-off event, in many cases assessments in adult social work usually lead to some form of care or support plan.

Assessments involve a range of skills including communication, information gathering, interviewing and observation, analysis and decision making. It is argued that social workers carrying out an assessment should aim to exercise 'reflection in action' (Shön, 1983) which is the ability to reflect upon what they are doing whilst they are doing it. However, some argue that this is difficult to do in the moment. Nevertheless, there should always be critical reflection and evaluation after the event (Coulshed and Orme, 2012).

It is argued that assessments can be made person-centred through the process of 'co-production' – the principle that those who use a service are best placed to help design it (SCIE, 2013; Bosco et al., 2019). However, whether this is always possible in practice with all adult service users is open to debate (Scourfield, 2015). Nevertheless, the general principles that should be applied to assessments are that they are carried out in partnership with the person as far as possible; that they are person-centred, holistic and promote the person's wellbeing (Hood, 2016).

There are different reasons why a social worker might carry out an assessment with someone living with dementia. In England, it will most commonly be an assessment of needs under the Care Act 2014. However, this assessment might also involve the need for an assessment of mental capacity and/or a carer's assessment. The interactive Care Act 2014 assessment and eligibility process map produced online by SCIE (2015) provides a good overview of the stages and processes in respect of the different assessments and the way they interrelate. (See www.scie.org. uk/care-act-2014/assessment-and-eligibility/process-map/.)

## Assessment with people living with dementia

It is pertinent to highlight that nearly all social work practice with people with dementia takes place in an organisational context where there are prescribed assessment formats and guidelines to be followed in what information is sought and for what purpose (Symonds et al., 2020). Social work assessments are often part of a more comprehensive multi-disciplinary assessment. The focus here, therefore, is *how* to carry out such assessments in ways that promote good person-centred dementia care and do not become too process-focused and disempowering as a consequence (Symonds et al., 2020). In reality, many assessments are iterative, dynamic and do not necessarily fit into discrete stages. However, for the purposes of this discussion, it is helpful to break the assessment task down into key components that need to be accomplished. These are pre-engagement preparation; engaging with the person and their support network; gathering information both *from* them and *about* them in regard to their situation – primarily through interviewing and observation; discussing preferred outcomes and agreeing a plan of action. In nearly all cases, information gathering would also extend to contacting other stakeholders such as health and housing professionals, as well as from the person's own case record if there is one.

## Pre-engagement preparation. Look out for labels

It is good practice to prepare well for meeting with the person. This involves critically examining the referral for what is being stated by the referrer and what is being requested. As explained earlier, information in referrals shape how the person is constructed and can suggest ready-made solutions. This is why referrals need to be read critically for depersonalising labels or other reductive 'blanket' descriptions such as 'challenging', 'aggressive', 'wanders' and so on. Stokes (2000) has demonstrated that when these behaviours occur, they always have something behind them which tells you more about the person's specific physical and emotional needs. In this respect, it is useful to contact referrers to obtain a fuller picture wherever possible. It is also useful to gather information from other people who know the person either personally or professionally. Although, in order to make an assessment person-centred it is important to avoid allowing others to define the person's needs and wants without input from the person themselves (Symonds et al., 2020).

It is important to find out at the start how the person likes to be called. Names are important. As Killick and Allan (2001) say 'using someone's name can be seen as a shortened way of respecting their personhood' (p. 246). However, only if it is the correct name. Someone's official name is not necessarily the name they like to be called by. Agency records should also be checked for previous involvements and to see whether there is a discernible pattern in previous referrals and interventions. Although this preparation can avoid the need for the person and their carer to repeat information already given, it is worth checking key information for accuracy and to gain a current perspective on what might be a recurrent issue or problem.

It is useful to establish what type of dementia the person has (see Chapter 2). This is not in order to offer medical opinions, but because Care Act guidance (Department of Health, 2014) requires practitioners to have the 'right skills and knowledge' to carry out an assessment (para. 6.3). Furthermore, knowing the basic features of different types of dementia can help build a relationship of trust as well as provide some insight into what the person is experiencing. So, for example, the person might say 'I've been told I've got vascular dementia – do you know what that is?' Instead of responding with 'No I don't, what is it?' It is more reassuring for the person to be told 'Yes, I know it's caused by reduced blood flow to the brain. How is it affecting you?' Social workers can walk something of a tightrope in how much medical knowledge they acquire and how they use it. Most people are reassured when a social worker is familiar with their medical condition in general terms. However, everyone's experience is different and it is important for them to be treated as individuals. Therefore, the key to person-centred practice is to start off with the right mindset. This means collecting as much relevant information as possible but maintaining an open mind about what the issues are and what needs to be done. This lays the foundations for, rather than predetermines, what develops from meeting the person face-to-face.

## Engaging with the person and their support network

Each case is different and there is no general formulation that can be made about whether a person-centred assessment should involve seeing the person on their own or in the company of members of their support network. It depends on the individual situation. The person's degree of impairment is obviously an important factor to consider, as is their relationship with other participants. If the person asks to be seen on their own, that is their choice, but people can often find it difficult to express this. On the other hand, many people actually welcome the support of someone they know. It will usually come down to a matter of professional judgement based on the individual situation.

If there are serious concerns about the relationship between the person and those who are with them, it could become a matter of adult safeguarding and the proper procedures should be followed. However, whether a person is enabled to speak alone, is more often a question of allowing them to be free to give their own perspective. Most carers understand this when it is explained to them.

On the question of how to achieve person-centred practice in assessments, a study by Symonds et al. (2020) concluded:

> Person-centred practice appeared most achievable when the practitioner spent time getting to know the person; when they did this without reference to the assessment form; and when they involved family members in the person's plan, but in an ancillary way. In contrast, when person-centred practice was likely to be compromised, this was characterised in practitioners' accounts when they used 'chat' in an instrumental way for assessment purposes; when they used the assessment form to conduct the meeting; and when they involved family members as more authoritative sources of information than the person.
>
> *(p. 443)*

However the communication is structured, the purpose of social work assessment meetings is to find the answers to key questions. This involves gathering information on the person's strengths, needs, the problems they face, what resources they have at their disposal and what their preferred outcomes are.

## Strengths-based approach

The Care Act 2014 advocates a strengths-based approach to social work with adults. This approach was originally developed by Saleeby (1996) in adult mental health services but has come to be applied to other service user groups (Nelson-Becker et al., 2020). There are different ways that strength-based approaches can be practised (Pattoni, 2012). However, one of its basic principles is that:

> The focus of the helping process is upon consumer's (sic) strengths, interests and abilities; not upon their weakness, deficit or pathologies.
>
> *(Coulshed and Orme, 2012: 163)*

The Care Act 2014 guidance (Department of Health, 2014) talks about considering the person's strengths and capabilities but also advocates looking for strengths to utilise in the person's family, wider support systems, other networks and the community more generally.

The strengths-based approach has been criticised by some for being too individualistic, over-optimistic and lacking a clear evidence base. However, an evidence-based social work practice with dementia is beginning to emerge. For example,

McGovern (2015) found that social work practitioners can maximise their effectiveness with people with dementia by, amongst other things:

- working with affected families, instead of individuals
- focusing on quality of life rather than symptom remediation
- adopting a strengths perspective
- enhancing clients' non-verbal communication skills
- facilitating participation in meaningful joint activities

*(p. 418)*

Given the complexity of the challenges presented by living with dementia, taking a 'strength-based' approach will not magically obviate all the problems, especially as the disease progresses in the latter stages. There has to be a certain degree of realism. However, the important point is that identifying a person's assets and helping them to use these to promote their wellbeing is more constructive than adopting an approach that is negative, fatalistic and focuses purely on deficits. Case Study 5.1 provides examples of how assessment interviews can be made more strengths-based.

## Case Study 5.1:   Strengths-based questioning

The following extract is adapted from *Strengths-based Social Work with Older People: A UK Perspective* by Nelson-Becker et al. (2020) and, as well as setting out the underlying principles, provides some examples of strengths-based questioning.

Overall, the approach should protect the individual's independence, resilience, ability to make choices and wellbeing. In order to achieve these aims and work in a strengths-based way, the importance of relationships and meaningful conversations is also emphasised. Such conversations might include elemental questions to enable the identification of strengths over deficits through the use of open language that does not privilege problems. Examples of such questions are:

- What does a good day look like for you?
- How do you spend your time?
- What matters most to you in life?
- Who is important to you?
- What kind of support do you receive?
- What has worked well for you previously
- What is going well for you now?
- What do you hope for? Why do you wake up each day?

*(p. 336)*

The case study provides an indication of the sort of questions that can be used with people with dementia and their carers. They are open, look for positives and help build relationships in a person–centred way. They also form the basis for assessments in which the person and their carers play as active a part as possible in formulating a suitable care and support plan. The degree to which the person can meaningfully participate will depend on how the disease is affecting them. However, even if they cannot answer the questions personally, these are the type of questions to which social workers should be seeking answers.

## Assessing and managing risks

Assessing and managing risk is an important part of social work with people with dementia. The loss of cognitive functions can lead to situations that compromise living independently and safely. For example, the person might forget to turn off the oven or other electrical equipment in the home or they might have episodes of confusion and disorientation when outside. This can be made worse by impaired communication. Diminished cognitive abilities can make someone more vulnerable to being exploited by unscrupulous others. Hearing, visual and physical impairments can also present risks to someone with dementia. They might be more unsteady and prone to falling for example. Therefore, overall, there are many potential risks that can come with the experience of living with dementia. The various risks attached to living with dementia can not only cause anxiety, concern and indecision for the person and their families but also for the professionals involved which, itself, can impact on decision making (Manthorpe, 2004). Because there is a subjective dimension to risk, reaching an agreement about how to proceed can present difficulties. For all of these reasons, it is useful to take an approach for assessing and managing risk that is both structured and defendable.

Partly because of the attitudes towards dementia discussed in Chapter 1, traditional approaches to risk management for people living with it have been overly cautious and risk-averse. This has often been to the point that the person's life has been diminished as much by the overprotective risk management measures as by dementia itself (Manthorpe, 2004; Department of Health, 2010b). As a consequence, official guidance now talks about 'risk enablement' and 'positive risk management' (Department of Health, 2010b). The guidance, *Nothing Ventured Nothing Gained*, explains it thus:

> Risk enablement is based on the idea that the process of measuring risk involves balancing the positive benefits from taking risks against the negative effects of attempting to avoid risk altogether. For example, the risk of getting lost if a person with dementia goes out unaccompanied needs to be set against the possible risks of boredom and frustration from remaining inside.
>
> *(Department of Health, 2010b: 8)*

The guidance *Nothing Ventured Nothing Gained* (Department of Health, 2010b) was written by Jill Manthorpe and Jo Moriarty with the principles of promoting independence and maximising risk and minimising restraint in mind. It includes a risk enablement framework that organisations can tailor to 'suit their own local circumstances' (p. 43). The framework has four steps:

1    Understanding the person's needs.
2    Understanding the impact of risks on the person.
3    Enabling and managing risk.
4    Risk planning.

Each step should be followed with the maximum involvement possible from the person. However, much as the principle of participation is important, the person's perspective alone cannot always be the deciding factor, as they might not be in the best position to understand the impacts of certain risk factors. It is good practice to seek the opinions of other professionals involved (Department of Health, 2015b). In fact, Hughes and Baldwin (2006) argue that it is actually a moral matter that the points of view of *all* the relevant people involved are taken into consideration. This particularly means carers and family members but includes anyone who might experience some form of harm if any risks are not managed properly. They call this the ethics of 'perspectivism' (p. 83).

Someone's mental capacity will obviously be a factor in determining how much they understand about the risks involved in any situation and what the likely impact will be of any risks identified (Smethurst, Robson and Killner, 2013). Therefore, assessing risk requires taking the person's mental capacity into account as well as understanding them in both their physical and their social context. This involves not only communicating with the person but also with those in their network. As Manthorpe (2004) says, risks need to be 'explored through discussions with people with dementia, their carers and a range of practitioners' (p. 148). The complexities and uncertainties surrounding many risk decisions in respect of people with dementia mean that there is often no simple, 'right' decision. In the context of uncertainty, it has been argued that professionals should aim to work towards risk decisions that are 'defendable' (Smethurst, Robson and Killner, 2013: 213). This means that practitioners should be able to demonstrate that:

- Reliable assessment methods were used.
- Appropriate information was collected from all relevant sources and evaluated thoroughly.
- Decisions were recorded and reasons given.
- Agency policies and national guidelines were followed.

In addition, professional judgement needs to be exercised in line with the principles of promoting person-centredness, empowerment and wellbeing. As discussed, *Nothing Ventured Nothing Gained* provided a broad framework for risk assessment, but there is no single risk assessment tool or format which will help decide exactly what to do in a particular individual's specific circumstances. However, Figure 5.1 shows a model adapted from Titterton (2005) that provides a suitable structure and would form the basis for defendable risk decisions.

*Identify the nature of each risk activity*
1 Identify the risk in discussion with all involved. Identify different points of view.
2 Specify the risk decision to be made (don't be too general or too vague)
  Be clear about:
  • what particular concerns you think makes this activity risky – what might go wrong?
  • what might people say should have been anticipated if things go wrong?
  • what are the benefits for the person if no action is taken?

*Identify where and when the risk activity will occur*
1 Identify the location(s) in which the risks will be incurred (e.g. in the street, the home, the kitchen, on transport, etc.)
2 Specify the timescale within which the risk activity is to take place.

*Identify possible outcomes/benefits and disadvantages*
1 List advantages and benefits from taking the risk for:
  • the individual,
  • family and friends,
  • other people
  • the service.
2 List disadvantages and possible harms which might arise for:
  • the individual,
  • family and friends,
  • other people
  • the service.
3 Include any opportunities that might be gained or lost.
4 Assign values placed on each of the benefits and harms by:
  • the individual,
  • carers
  • the assessor.
  In other words what importance is attached to each of the identified benefits and harms according to the main parties to the risk decision?

*Estimate likelihood of risk*
1 Estimate the likelihood of each type of harm within the specified time frame to:
  • the individual,
  • family and friends,
  • other people
  • your service and other agencies.
2 Decide on the likelihood of each harm within the specified time frame to see if it is:
  (a) unlikely to happen,
  (b) may happen or
  (c) very likely to happen.

Adapted from Titterton (2005)

**FIGURE 5.1** Key steps in risk assessment

The model of risk assessment in Figure 5.1 does not need to be adopted too rigidly. It can be tailored to suit particular situations. However, it tries to 'unpack' the risk(s) as fully as possible and aims to achieve decisions about risks that are made logically and systematically. It also tries to ensure that decisions are specific and taken on a risk-by-risk basis. To maintain person-centredness, it is important that 'blanket' decisions based on generalisations about dementia are avoided (Clarke et al., 2011). Therefore, if it is said, for example, that it is far too risky for someone with dementia to be living in their own house, the model provides a process with which to analyse that kind of judgement in detail. Significantly, it also requires the assessor to think about and declare their own position, which is important from the point of view of taking professional responsibility and of practising with transparency.

## Risk management/risk mitigation/risk enablement

For some, the phrase 'risk management' suggests that risk can be eliminated altogether – which, in most cases, is neither possible or desirable. Risk enablement is about enabling a person with dementia to take part in an activity or do something in ways that mitigate the risk to acceptable levels but still respects their choices and promotes their quality of life (Department of Health, 2010b). This can only really be done by getting to know the person and those around them which, in turn, can only be achieved through good communication and sharing of information about risks (Clarke et al., 2011). Risk enablement requires that the strengths that each person with dementia possesses are recognised and that whatever abilities that he or she has retained are built upon where possible (Department of Health, 2010b: 8). So, for example, if someone with memory problems is still capable of understanding a calendar or consulting a diary, then these methods should be used to provide appropriate reminders and memory prompts to ensure that their day runs smoothly. The calendar or diary might need to be made more conspicuous and written more clearly but is about exploiting a skill or habit that a person already had in order to compensate for the inability to retain as much information as before. There is a range of assistive technology and other services that can help in this respect which is discussed in more detail in Chapter 6.

## Activity 5.2: Dementia and driving

George is 72 and has just been told by the doctors that he is in the first stages of Alzheimer's disease. He has been driving since he was 17. He even passed an advanced driving test when he was working as a courier earlier in his life. George likes driving. It gives him pleasure and it also helps him feel useful. His wife Jill cannot drive, so George drives them both everywhere, including to the shops, the doctors and so on. He feels that he is still safe to drive and there is very little or no risk at present. However, Jill is worried that he won't be safe because he has started having episodes of confusion. She definitely thinks there are some risks to George continuing to drive. Their daughter is determined that George should give up completely now, just in case he has an accident. She thinks it is just too risky. They ask you, as their social worker, what should they do?

1   After giving your initial thoughts, read the section on Driving and Dementia on the Alzheimer's Society website: www.alzheimers.org.uk/get-support/ staying-independent/driving-dementia#content-start

2   You should look at other research and opinion on this issue, such as the 'Driving, memory loss and dementia' blog on the NHS England website: www.england.nhs.uk/blog/driving-memory-loss-and-dementia written by Burns and McShane, two eminent psychiatrists of old age.

3   What were your initial reactions to George's situation? How, were they changed by reading the information and how would you advise George and Jill about the risks involved?

Activity 5.2 illustrates several key points in respect of assessing and managing risks associated with dementia. First, it underlines that it is a complex activity and can often be a contested area. Risk is felt subjectively and everyone will not share the same perspective. Risks are usually dynamic – they change over time and according to different circumstances. Information from the links states that UK law requires George to inform the licensing authority about his diagnosis, but that he does not necessarily have to give up driving. So the law on its own will not necessarily help in making decisions about how to manage risk. There is advice available on the links to help George to continue to drive safely. However, although George might be confident and be prepared to take the risk, an activity like driving can, potentially, be seriously harmful to others if something went wrong. Risk decisions can affect many people and not just the person with dementia. In George's situation, a balance needs to be struck between competing interests. George and his family would also benefit from short, medium and long-term planning. The risk needs to be closely monitored and plans adapted accordingly. The focus of much of the work might be, for example, ensuring that George is given every assistance in continuing to drive safely for the time being, but that he and Jill should be helped to prepare to make alternative provisions for their transport needs in the future. The activity also raises issues about the loss of independence, role and identity for George. More will be discussed about loss as an important concept in social work practice with dementia later in the chapter.

## Supporting people living with dementia to be involved in adult safeguarding enquiries

Both risk assessments and risk management form an important part of the adult safeguarding process. Section 42 of the Care Act 2014 requires local authorities in England to instigate a safeguarding enquiry when there are indications of abuse or neglect in relation to an adult with care and support needs who is at risk and is unable to protect themselves because of those needs. The diagnosis of dementia on its own does not mean that everyone living with dementia will come into the category, although many will, and it has been found that older adults living with dementia are at greater risk of abuse and neglect than those without a diagnosis (Fang and Yan, 2018).

The purpose of a safeguarding enquiry is to decide what action is needed to help and protect the adult. Its aims are to:

•   establish the facts about an incident or allegation;

- ascertain the adult's views and wishes on what they want as an outcome from the enquiry;
- assess the needs of the adult for protection, support and redress and how they might be met;
- protect the adult from the abuse and neglect, as the adult wishes;
- establish if any other person is at risk of harm;
- make decisions as to what follow-up actions should be taken with regard to the person or organisation responsible for the abuse or neglect and
- enable the adult to achieve resolution and recovery.

Once an enquiry has been carried out the findings are used to decide whether abuse or neglect has taken place and whether the adult at risk needs a protection plan. This is a set of arrangements that are required to keep the person safe. The Department of Health and Social Care (2021) has produced guidance on how to support people living with dementia to be involved in adult safeguarding enquiries. Informed by *Making Safeguarding Personal* (LGA, 2014), it is based on a human rights approach and the FRIEDA principles discussed in earlier chapters, namely Fairness, Respect, Equality, Identity, Dignity and Autonomy. The guidance recommends that:

> When a safeguarding enquiry is made, practitioners must consider how the person in question views the alleged abuse or neglect and should ensure that they are central to decision-making. Such decisions involve thinking about risk and making proportionate judgements about it.
>
> *(Department of Health and Social Care, 2021: 5)*

This underlines that safeguarding practice with people with dementia requires good communication, empathy and relationship-building skills, in fact, the full skillset required for person-centred dementia care. In relation to taking a strengths-based approach, the guidance refers to a practice tool developed by Stanley (2016) based on the 'signs of safety' framework used in children's safeguarding. This framework is about identifying what is going well for the person as much as it is about identifying what is threatening their safety. These approaches all underline a shift in how people with dementia in regarded in adult social care. They are no longer constructed one-dimensionally as passive and tragic victims to be 'done to' and looked after for their own good. Instead, they are regarded first and foremost as 'people' with rights, strengths, coping skills, resilience and feelings. People to be worked *with*, even when at their most vulnerable.

## Working with carers

Working with family and other carers is a very important part of social work practice with people with dementia (Department of Health, 2015b). However, this area of practice is not without considerable complexity and requires empathy, judgement, 'diplomacy' and a good knowledge of relevant information, such as legal entitlements, benefits, health services, support services and so on. There are many potential issues to consider when working with carers. Carers are often valuable sources of care and support for the person and they usually have much useful information about the person's past life and their current situation with which to inform assessment and care planning (Whitlach, 2014). They also have their own emotional, physical and social needs. Their agenda and values can sometimes be in conflict with that of the person for whom they are caring and with other people in the person's network (Whitlach, 2014). Younger family members can also have the additional stress of worrying about whether they, too, will develop dementia (Jarvik et al., 2008). Family carers can experience strong feelings of grief as the person's disease progresses, particularly towards the end of life stages (Zarit and Zarit, 2014).

Not only can the circumstances, role and attitudes of carers change over time so can the relationship between carers and social care professionals (Twigg and Atkin, 1994). For example, a carer who refuses help initially might soon not only require it but also want to be free completely of the caring role. Therefore, it is unhelpful to attach labels to carers such as 'independent' and 'refuses any help'. Caring relationships are dynamic and can change quickly.

People with dementia experience a relatively high incidence of abuse from carers (Cooper et al., 2009). This is for various reasons, but the challenges presented by caring for someone with dementia and the associated carer stress are major factors (Zarit and Zarit, 2014). Studies have indicated when the person with dementia has depression, sleep disturbance or wandering behaviour this can be especially stressful for carers (Adams and Manthorpe, 2003). It can also be stressful having to make 'best interests' decisions for the other person. Medical and other important life decisions such as whether someone should be moved to a care home can be complex and very consequential for all parties involved.

A percentage of carers also report being abused by the person with dementia (Adams and Manthorpe, 2003). In the later stages of dementia, some people will develop behavioural and psychological symptoms of dementia. These include paranoia and agitated and aggressive behaviours such as shouting, screaming, verbal abuse, accusations and, sometimes, physical abuse (NHS, n.d.). For these and other reasons, carers can often have very mixed feelings towards the person for whom they are caring and these feelings can change over time as the person's disease deteriorates. Therefore, whilst the focus of social work with people with dementia should necessarily be person-centred – on the person with dementia – the needs and situations of their carers must also be attended to. This underlines the need for a practice that is person-centred and strengths-based but is also relationship-based and systemic in its approach. From their research, Adams and Manthorpe (2003) provide some useful insights into the carer–recipient relationship. They state that:

> Interpersonal relationships between people with dementia and their carers have been found to be characterized by more hostility and less affection than relationships between carers and people with other mental health problems.

Many carers report difficulties arising from a change in relationship with the person, which is often associated with the 'loss' of the person as previously known, this being caused by the cognitive and personality changes associated with dementia. Carers who are spouses have been found to exhibit more distress than non-spouse carers which may be partly the result of the alteration in a longstanding relationship and intimacy.

*(p. 193)*

Although the research was carried out several years ago, there is no reason to believe that most, if not all, of what they say remains relevant. As much as anything, it underlines the importance of understanding the impact of loss and change in such relationships.

## Primary and secondary stressors in caregiving relationships

Examining 'carer–care recipient' stress in more depth led Zarit and Zarit (2014) to conclude that there are 'primary' and 'secondary' stressors. Primary stressors are related directly to the illness and secondary stressors are indirectly related. Primary caregiving stressors fall into three categories:

- Changes in the person's cognition and abilities.
- Behavioural and emotional changes.
- Changes in the relationship between the carer and the person with dementia, including a sense of loss (p. 178).

Obviously the exact changes depend on the individual and the type of dementia they have. People often live together in multiple family and social systems, sometimes under the same roof, but not necessarily so. Change in one person will have an impact on other people in that system. However, this might not always be immediately observable. So, for example, a daughter who lives 50 miles from her parent with dementia might not only visit more often once the diagnosis is made, they also might put off applying for a job promotion that involves moving to a different part of the country and would make visiting more difficult. This decision, in turn, might have 'knock on' effects on her family and other systems. This underlines the need to understand the impact of secondary stressors as much as primary ones. It also highlights the interconnectedness and interdependency between people and the importance of taking a systems approach to social work practice (Teater, 2014).

Secondary stressors include:

- The impact of caring on the carer's usual activities, including work and leisure.
- Conflict or strain in family relationships and friendships.
- Economic strains (p. 180).

Again, these cannot be generalised. However, in addition to the physical and emotional costs of caring, the financial costs must not be forgotten. This is not just the cost of care itself but also the loss of the contribution from the person with dementia, if they can no longer work, and also the loss of earnings of caregivers who have given up their own employment in order to care (Carers UK, 2012; Marie Curie, 2015). Economic strain often brings or adds to the emotional strain of caring. Family members can often be in conflict with each other not only about how to manage the person's care but also how to manage the costs of care (Zarit and Zarit, 2014).

The following practice tips are offered for working with family and informal caregivers:

- First, there is no universal 'carer' and no single, typical carer–recipient relationship. The impact of caring and the issues which an individual carer or family member might be struggling with cannot be assumed. This would particularly apply to people and carers from minority LGBT and BAME communities. Carers should therefore not be encouraged to behave in ways that do not suit their particular relationships or that are culturally inappropriate.
- Do not assume that the presence of a spouse or other family member in someone's living environment automatically makes them a 'carer'. Neither their willingness nor their competence to care for that person should be taken for granted.
- Not everyone in a caregiving or supporting role likes to be called a 'carer'.
- However, if they are performing the role they should still be offered a Carer's Assessment (Department of Health, 2014). If it is declined this choice should be recorded.
- The process of the assessment itself can be useful for the carer to make sense of their experiences and explore their own needs and options. Even if it does not lead to services, it can help them to disentangle their feelings about themselves from their feelings about the person for whom they are caring and about their changing relationship.
- Discuss carers' needs and issues in a separate conversation, especially when exploring the sustainability of the caring role.
- Because of possible conflicts of interest, person-centred care for the person and tailored support for the carer can be better promoted by having a separate worker or advocate for the carer.
- The caregiving–recipient relationship is dynamic. It changes over time and according to changing circumstances. Keep the situation under review.
- Think and practise systemically. The impact of an individual living with dementia will usually impact on others in their networks, which, in turn, will impact on the person with dementia.
- Take a strengths-based approach but do not allow this to lead to an overestimation of a carer's coping skills and resilience. A strengths-based approach should not be seen as an opportunity to overload responsibilities onto people who, out of feelings of obligation and guilt, might feel unable to challenge this.
- Anticipate the need for a wide range of information and be prepared to provide it in different formats depending on the needs of the carer.

- Develop and maintain knowledge about a range of relevant local and national services, including specific stress-relieving services for carers.
- Support groups and other group facilities are not for everyone. Consider and provide alternative support opportunities. This is where it is useful to provide information about Personal Budgets.
- The science in respect of whether certain types of dementia are hereditary and what the risk factors are is complex and incomplete. Social workers should signpost family members worrying about these types of issues to a medical specialist for counselling.

## The life course, change and loss

Theories of the life course, loss and change are important areas of knowledge for all branches of social work (BASW, 2018). In the study of adult development, life course theories have tended to replace traditional stage theories because they take into account more variables and more contextual factors in understanding how people's lives develop over the whole life course (Settersten and Hendricks, 2003). Life course theories are based on the broad assumption that our lives are shaped by age, social structures and historical change (Elder and Johnson, 2003). In addition to factors such as our gender, class and ethnicity, life course theory flags the importance of other factors that shape our development. These are briefly discussed in the sections that follow. As understanding someone's life trajectory is one of the foundations for person-centred practice with people with dementia, identifying and understanding the factors that help shape their particular life trajectories is important.

### Life-span development

People develop biologically, socially, and psychologically over their whole lifetime and not just in their childhood years. Although situations encountered in adult-hood are shaped by earlier life experiences and the meanings attached to them, they are not pre-determined. See the 'Agency' section.

### Time and place

Where and when we are born and brought up is important. For example, the life of a 65-year-old man born in London in the 1950s will differ from a 65-year woman born and brought up in Jamaica and who moved to Birmingham in the 1970s, even though they are exactly the same age. Not only are they of a different gender, but they were also born into different socio-historical, geographical and cultural environments. Similarly, the life of an 80-year-old man born in London in the 1930s will be different from that of a 65-year-old man. They are the same gender and were brought up in broadly the same geographical environment but the social, economic and cultural environment in which they grew up will differ in many important ways.

## Timing

The concept of time here refers to an individual's own life chronology rather than the historical and cultural times in which they were born, brought up and live in. So, for example, two 40-year-old women might be from the same class background and from the same part of town. However, one might have had her first child at the age of 17, left school and put off continuing her education until she was 33. The other might have gone to university at 18, pursued a career and had her first child at the age of 36. This would make for two quite different life trajectories.

## Agency

Whatever circumstances they are born into and what upbringing they have, people are always, to some degree, 'agentic'. This does not mean that we are completely free to choose whatever life we want. Important structural factors such as class, gender, race and age need to be taken into account. However, it does mean that we make choices that influence the shape of their lives to some extent. People exercise their agency in different ways and according to different values. For example, some focus on the 'here and now' whilst others focus on long-term goals. Some of our decisions are selfish, others more altruistic. Personality traits and values play an important part in how agency is expressed.

## Linked lives

We are social beings. Most people's lives are lived interdependently and reflect shared cultural and socio-historical influences. Our various social relationships and the common experiences that come with them help provide a common context with which we interpret life events.

This brief summary has aimed to show the relevance of life course theories to dementia social work. Compared to stage theories, they factor in many variables into understanding how someone's life develops and how that person has developed into who they are. Taking this approach helps situate the person in their fullest possible context and to see them as three-dimensional people whose life stories encompass various changes and transitions (Bywaters, 2007).

Another reason for taking a life course approach is that people with dementia make sense of what is happening to them in the here and now by reference to experiences they have had in the past (Brooker, 2007). As McColgan (2004) found in her research with nursing home residents, telling stories about their past helped people with dementia to reconstruct their identity and make sense of the present. Knowledge of someone's life course can therefore help with life story and life review work, which has proved a helpful intervention for many people living with dementia (Thompson, 2011). The key to understanding what seem to be problematic behaviours in someone's present life can often come from knowledge of their life story (Stokes, 2000). Lastly, having a reasonable understanding of the key elements and changes in someone's life trajectory can help with 'best interests' decisions if they no longer have the capacity to make important life decisions for themselves.

## Loss

Ideas about change and loss in the life course also need to avoid over-simplistic models that do not take enough account of individual and cultural differences. For example, for many years, the five-stage model of grief (denial, anger, bargaining, depression and acceptance) proposed by Kübler-Ross (1989) was more or less accepted as universally applicable. However, it has subsequently been critiqued for, amongst other things, lacking a properly scientific evidence base and being too rigid and deterministic (Konigsberg, 2011). This does not mean that all of Kübler-Ross's ideas need to be rejected, particularly about the symptoms of grief, but it does mean that alternative theories of loss should be explored for what they can contribute. For example, the dual-process model (Stroebe and Schut, 1999) suggests that grief operates in that ways that are both loss-oriented and restoration-oriented. People switch back and forth between them in ways that meet their needs. The dual-process model does not make the assumption that it is necessarily 'healthy' or 'natural' to respond to loss by 'working through' a set series of emotions. Rather than label people as being 'in denial', it states that it can be helpful to ignore your emotions, get on with things and distract yourself from your grief by engaging in everyday and future-orientated activities. Again, it is useful not to cling to a single model of loss and grief because people are different and react to and cope with losses in their own different ways. They are not necessarily behaving wrongly if they do not display certain stereotyped notions of what grief reactions should be. Social work practice around people experiencing losses and grieving should not be about encouraging people to feel in certain ways or try to interpret their feelings for them. Sometimes the best thing to do is to accept that loss and suffering are part of life and to bear witness to what the person is going through and allow them to make sense of what is going on in their own way. This means 'being' with the person (physically and emotionally) and giving them space rather than doing something which is designed to mitigate or psychologise any feelings that they might be experiencing.

## Activity 5.3: Loss and change

- What changes and losses might a person in the first stages of Alzheimer's be experiencing? How might this make them feel? What might they need?
- What changes and losses might a spouse of a person with Alzheimer's be experiencing? How might this make them feel? What might they need?

Activity 5.3 can only be answered in general terms. You would need to know a lot more about the person in question to answer the questions satisfactorily. This is one of the key learning points of the activity – we can formulate our own ideas but we must allow for individual differences. However, activity was designed to prompt reflection that when someone develops dementia, not only do various changes and losses happen in their lives, but also others around them also experience their own changes and losses. As was discussed in relation to primary and secondary stressors, a dynamic interrelationship exists between different parts of the person's family and other networks and the effects of some losses are more observable than others.

A reasonable response to the questions would be to suggest that, in those circumstances, people might have feelings of uncertainty, confusion and anxiety. There can be many losses associated with dementia; for example, loss of memory, loss of sense of place, loss of physical capabilities, loss of job, loss of role and even loss of self. Dementia can bring about multiple, overlapping losses. However, unlike the loss when someone dies, many of the losses that can accompany dementia lack the same finality of a single event such as death. To be able to practise social work with empathy, it is useful to have an understanding of the concept of 'ambiguous loss'.

## Ambiguous loss

The concept of ambiguous loss was developed in the 1970s by Boss who studied the reactions of families of soldiers missing in action. The soldiers were missing but it was not known whether they were dead, captured or hiding and might therefore return. For their families, the lack of finality complicated the process of dealing with the loss. From that study, the concept of ambiguous loss has been shown to have broader applications beyond when the person is physically missing. Boss and Yeats (2014) explain that:

> Ambiguous loss is a loss that remains unclear and without resolution. It has no closure or finality because the loss is ongoing. There are two types of ambiguous loss. . . . The second type of ambiguous loss is psychological: a loved one is physically present but psychologically absent due, for example, to memory loss and cognitive impairment, as a result of dementia from Alzheimer's disease or one of the over 50 other diseases or injuries that cause dementia.
>
> (p. 64)

Subsequently, others have highlighted the relevance of ambiguous loss to understanding dementia grief better. It is similar to anticipatory loss which refers to the mourning that begins to take place when a someone is expected to die. However, it is more complicated by the nature of dementia itself. Blandin and Pepin (2017) explain that this is because dementia has losses that 'are unstable and fluctuating, evading finality and resolution' (p. 3). With dementia, some of the ambiguous loss is connected to the unpredictable trajectory of the disease itself. No one can be sure exactly how it will develop, at what pace and what its precise impact will be. There are many potential ambiguous losses associated with dementia. Blandin and Pepin (2017) give examples where the impact of dementia is such that family members can experience an [ambiguous] loss of hope that past conflicts with the person with dementia can be reconciled in the future. Ambiguous loss can also be experienced in relation to ideas and expectations about what the future holds. Blandin and Pepin (2017) say that ambiguous loss is rarely recognised by family members themselves or by others. The lack of resolution from ambiguous losses associated with dementia can last for years with the final resolution of grief only occurring once the person has physically died.

This raises questions about how to help people deal with ambiguous loss. Boss and Yeats (2014) suggest a six-point framework that helps manage the feelings associated with it. Being aware of the concept is the first step but much of it is about recognising the reality of the situation and being prepared to make psychological adjustments to the changes that are happening. The points are as follows.

## Naming the problem and finding meaning

It is useful to explain to people that the feelings that they are experiencing are probably due to 'ambiguous loss' and that it is a difficult kind of loss to deal with because there is no possibility of resolution. As Boss and Yeats (2014: 68) say, 'once people have a name for what is bothering them, they can begin the coping process'. They can begin to make better sense of the situation, which is often done by sharing their feelings with others affected.

## Normalising ambivalence

This is about accepting that, with ambiguous loss, it is normal to have conflicted feelings. Talking about them helps to manage and normalise the ambivalence.

## Tempering mastery

This means that it needs to be accepted that it is nobody's fault that someone close is being 'lost' to dementia, and more to the point, much of the time, there is very little that can be done to change (or 'master') the situation. Accepting this does not necessarily eliminate all negative feelings but it can help people manage some of those feelings, such as guilt, self-blame and frustration. Boss and Yeats report that when someone finds it difficult to master the ambiguity surrounding a loss, they encourage them to balance their feelings of helplessness with 'internal self-mastery'. They found that engaging in activities like meditation, prayer, mindfulness, playing music and exercise are useful in this respect. 'Tempering mastery' is about controlling the things you can control and not 'beating yourself up' about those that you cannot.

## Redefining relationships and reconstructing identity

Boss and Yeats suggest that in order to develop resilience it is helpful to redefine personal relationships. This involves recognising that certain aspects of the relationship are lost. It also means being more flexible with the boundaries, roles and rules of the 'old' relationship. Ways of functioning together need to be adapted to accommodate the losses experienced. This needs to be an ongoing process.

### Revising attachment to the missing person

Revising attachment means grieving for what and who has been lost whilst celebrating what remains. Boss and Yeats also say that this means making a point of being with people socially who can be fully present.

### Discover new hopes and dreams despite the pain of ambiguous loss

Boss and Yeats argue that the opportunity to build resilience is impeded by demanding an end to grief and suffering whilst the person is still alive. They say that people need to become more comfortable with the ambiguity and uncertainty and that, once they do, they are more free to discover new sources of hope. If possible, people should be encouraged to laugh at the absurdity of their ambiguous loss whilst also acknowledging the pain of it. If they can get to this point, they can free themselves up enough to create new options for hope.

There is not a solid evidence base to show that the six-point framework works for all people experiencing the ambiguous losses associated with dementia. It is not as structured or as researched as, say, cognitive behavioural therapy (CBT) where there is evidence to show that CBT is a useful intervention for caregivers of people with dementia (Kwon et al., 2017). However, what both approaches have in common is encouraging people to actively manage their cognitions and feelings and to look for positives in their situation. The social work role often does not allow much time to work therapeutically with either people with dementia or their carers. However, it is useful to incorporate key points from the aforementioned framework in discussions, even if it is confined to giving a name to the experience of ambiguous loss in order to enable individuals to make sense of the situation and find some psychological comfort.

## Conclusion

This chapter has set out the main contexts in which social work with people living with dementia and carers is practised, together with the principle tasks involved. There can be no doubt that all social work practice with dementia is complex because of the nature of the disease and the impact it has on people's lives. Although the primary focus in the chapter has been on communication, observation, assessment and empathy skills, social workers need to employ the full range of social work skills required when working in a multi-disciplinary context. This would include skills in inter-professional working, networking and advocacy. The chapter has stressed the importance of being able to practise using person-centred, strengths-based and systemic approaches. In addition, it has highlighted the ability to both understand the needs of and provide support to carers. The final section discussed the usefulness of being able to apply theories of the life course, change and loss as an aid to both developing empathy and person-centred practice. Underpinning everything is the skill of critical reflection which, amongst other things, provides a necessary guard against lapsing into stereotyped thinking and failing to recognise the individual person in this important area of social work practice.

## Further reading

Department of Health (2015). *A Manual for Good Social Work Practice Supporting Adults Who Have Dementia*. London: DH Publications.

The title is self-explanatory. It is a relatively brief set of guidelines, but the chapters include, 'person-centred approach', 'working with carers', 'advocating', 'challenging' as well as links to resources.

Department of Health and Social Care (2021). *Supporting People Living with Dementia to Be Involved in Adult Safeguarding Enquiries*. London: Department of Health and Social Care/ University of Bath.

Again, the title is self-explanatory. This guidance is divided into two parts: 'evidence summary' and 'suggestions for good practice'. There is also a useful list of references.

Skills for Care (2015/2018). *Dementia Core Skills Education and Training Framework*. London: Skills for Care, Skills for Health and Health Education England.

Although aimed primarily at educators, this is a useful document for practitioners in the social care workforce to access because it contains a wide range of references on the skills and knowledge required to practise good dementia care.

# 6

# DEMENTIA CARE AND SUPPORT SERVICES

By the end of this chapter, you should have an understanding of:

- The different services available to support people living with dementia and their carers.

## Introduction

Social work is just one of a wide range of care and support services that are available to meet the needs of people living with dementia and their carers in the UK. However, the needs of people living with dementia are many and diverse. In order to provide a service that is person centred and holistic, social workers need to be aware of what other services are available, how these services are accessed, what purposes they serve and what needs they meet. Therefore, the central goal of this chapter is to illustrate the range of potential services available to people with dementia and their carers. It aims to encourage an approach to social work practice that actively seeks out as many different appropriate services and interventions as possible. Providing information and advice about relevant services to people who might need or want them is a core task of social work. It will help the person with dementia and their carers have more choice over how they are supported and it will enhance the possibility of their receiving more personalised care and support services.

Unfortunately, services are not uniformly distributed or organised across the UK and there can be significant local variations in what is available, as well as how services are named and accessed. Also, services are changing all the time, so for the most up to date and accurate information on local services readers are advised to do their own research. Nevertheless, this chapter will provide an illustration of the types of statutory, voluntary and private services that are currently available. The different services and organisations discussed in this chapter are mainly from England and

DOI: 10.4324/9781003191667-7

around the countries of the UK. However, mostly they are indicative of services that are now available or becoming available for people with dementia internationally.

## Health services

In the UK, the main provider of health services is the NHS which operates on three levels; primary, secondary and tertiary. As their disease progresses people with dementia will almost certainly use primary and secondary health care services and, in some cases, might well use services at all three levels.

### *Primary health care*

Primary health care is the first point of contact for health care for most people. Primary health care refers to services that can be accessed directly. These include GPs, community pharmacists, optometry services, dentists and services attached to health centres and GP surgeries such as heart and asthma nurses. The chances are that most people who are referred for social work services are already involved with at least one primary health service – usually their GP. If, during their practice, social workers meet anyone who is worried that either they or a member of their family has dementia and they have not consulted their GP, they should be encouraged to do so. If, after examination, the GP believes that someone has some form of cognitive impairment, they usually refer them to a Memory Assessment Team/ Clinic or a dementia specialist for more specialist assessment. Some GP surgeries employ Dementia Care Coordinators whose role is to support and coordinate the care for individuals diagnosed with dementia and other cognitive impairments.

Some areas operate a Dementia Advisor Service whose role includes:

- helping people and their families understand the diagnosis of dementia,
- providing emotional support,
- providing advice to enable people to live well in their own home, including how to prevent falls and accidents,
- providing information about local and national support services, including local memory cafes and activity groups and
- referring on to health, voluntary and social care services based on assessment.

Access to a Dementia Advisor can either be by self-referral or, more commonly, by a referral from the person's GP or other community health and social care professional.

Admiral Nurses are specialist dementia nurses who work in different settings such as care homes, hospitals and hospices but can also be attached to GP surgeries (Dementia UK, n.d. b). They are qualified Registered Mental Nurses (RMNs) who have completed post registration courses in dementia care. They are funded primarily by the charity Dementia UK and not able to offer a comprehensive service across the whole of the UK. Local availability can be checked through the Dementia UK website www.dementiauk.org/get-support/find-an-admiral-nurse/.

However, they run a free Dementia helpline, so they can be contacted directly. A GP's referral is not necessary.

As experts in dementia care Admiral Nurses play more of an advisory and counselling role rather than a day-to-day, 'hands on' caring role. They are very useful in advising about skills and techniques to help manage any communication difficulties, psychological problems, co-morbidities, end of life or other difficult situations that a person with dementia or their carers might be experiencing.

## Secondary health care

A referral from a primary care practitioner (usually a GP) is required to access secondary health care. Secondary health care describes health services to which a person might be referred if they need to be seen by someone with more specialist knowledge about their condition, such as a hospital consultant. For people with dementia this will usually be a consultant neurologist whose specialism is the brain and nervous system or a psychiatrist who specialises in mental health and mental disorders. People over 65 might be referred to a geriatrician who specialises in the physical illnesses and disabilities of old age or a psychogeriatrician whose specialism is mental disorders in older people. Some people end up under the care of more than one consultant, especially if they have co-morbidities.

Apart from the branches of medicine outlined earlier, there are many other secondary health care services for people with dementia. These include speech and language therapy; physiotherapy, audiology (hearing), optometry (eyesight); podiatry (feet), dieticians and clinical psychology. Speech and language therapists can offer support through swallowing and speech exercises, dietary advice and changes to medication. Dietary advice is particularly important, as malnutrition is common in older people with dementia. As well as help with diet and nutrition, dieticians can also assist with the eating and swallowing difficulties that can come with dementia. The clinical psychologist role includes assessing memory and other cognitive skills. They also offer support to both the person with dementia and their carers with managing behavioural problems and mental difficulties such as anxiety or depression. Clinical psychologists can work in different settings. For example, they can be attached to health centres, hospitals or work as part of a multi-disciplinary community mental health team. Clinical psychologists also work in memory clinics which play an important role in assessing people suspected of having dementia.

## Memory clinics

Memory clinics (sometimes known as memory services) are not a designated dementia service as such, they assess all memory problems, some of which might have different causes. However, much of their work is concerned with helping to assess and diagnose dementia. They are a multi-disciplinary facility comprising medical and psychologically trained staff as well as nursing and other specialists.

Not all areas of the UK have access to a memory clinic and not all clinics are run by the NHS, some are privately run. Apart from psychological testing, memory clinics can perform detailed brain scans, for example, CT (computed tomography) or MRI scans (magnetic resonance imaging). The images are used to help diagnose of dementia and identify what type of dementia it is. As well as serving a diagnostic function, memory clinics offer psychosocial interventions such as CST, CBT and life story work (see also the section on psychological therapies in Chapter 4). They can also provide signposting to other services. Often this is done by Dementia Coordinators who also provide post-diagnostic support for people with a diagnosis of dementia and for their families and carers. Since they were first established in the 1980s referrals to memory clinics have been steadily rising and waiting times have been increasing (Dementia Statistics, 2021d). The high demand on their services is said to be a reason why memory clinics do not always provide enough support for people once they have been diagnosed. At the time of writing, this is an issue being researched by a Centre of Excellence funded by the Alzheimer's Society at Newcastle University in the UK.

As well as have an impact on mental functioning dementia can have an impact on a range of bodily functions. Two common problems experienced by people with dementia as it progresses are falls and incontinence. Specialist services have been developed in both of these areas.

## Continence

Most areas operate an NHS continence advisory service which is usually provided by a specialist nurse-led team whose function is to assess, treat and manage bladder and bowel problems that impact on the quality of someone's everyday life. It is quite common, for example, for people to 'manage' their urinary incontinence by drinking less which usually leads to dehydration. Apart from causing discomfort, embarrassment and inconvenience, incontinence can also lead to social withdrawal. Referrals to continence advisors are usually required by a GP, but services vary, so it is always worth checking what exactly is available locally and what the referral procedures are.

## Falls

Most areas also operate an NHS Falls Prevention Service which provides assessment, advice and exercise programmes for people (usually) aged 65 and over who are at risk of falling. The service aims to prevent falls and unnecessary admission to hospital by seeing people considered to be at risk of falling, providing advice and supporting them with a maintenance programme after rehabilitation. Although the factors related to increased fall risk in people with dementia are not fully understood, the Falls Prevention Service can offer practical ways of minimizing the risks. Access to this service is usually via the person's GP. But referral arrangements can vary according to location.

## Occupational therapy

Occupational therapy services do not just sit within the NHS, like physiotherapists they work across different health and social care services in both the statutory and non-statutory sectors. Referrals for occupational therapy can be made via the person's GP or another member of the local community healthcare team. Occupational therapists help people carry out the activities of daily life that dementia prevents them from doing. These include activities such as meal preparation, getting washed and dressed, moving around the home safely and engaging in social activities. Occupational therapists work with people with dementia and their carers in several different ways. They can advise people on what they can do to live as independently as possible, for example, by making changes around the home. They can advise on adaptations, equipment and assistive technology that can be purchased privately or loaned from health and social services (see the section on 'Technology enabled care' later in this chapter). An occupational therapist can improve safety in the home by providing advice on safety devices and alarms that are low cost or free and readily available. They can also provide advice on exercises that can help relieve anxiety and depression and demonstrate how to use reminiscence and life story work (see the section on psychological therapies in Chapter 4).

When carrying out assessments with people with dementia it is very useful for social workers to make sure that their GP knows about the various impacts the dementia is having on their lives and has linked them to the various specialist health services that are available locally. Some services will accept referrals from social workers and other professionals but it is always good practice to involve, or at least inform, the person's GP and, if there is one locally, their Dementia Care Coordinator or Dementia Adviser.

## Tertiary health care

Tertiary health care is the part of NHS provision which serves people with very complex or rare conditions. This usually takes place in a few specialist hospitals where the person receives highly specialised care performed by medical specialists using the most up to date research and procedures. Tertiary health care facilities are usually also research centres. To access tertiary health care a person would normally require a referral from a consultant in secondary health care.

An example of tertiary care for people with dementia is the University College London (UCL) Dementia Research Centre. The Dementia Research Centre hosts the Rare Dementia Support facility which is for people affected by, or at risk of, seven of the rare dementias. These are: FAD, young-onset Alzheimer's disease, FTD, familial FTD, posterior cortical atrophy, primary progressive aphasia and Lewy body dementia. Much of the work of the Dementia Research Centre is about identifying and understanding the rare dementias better, developing ways to improve diagnosis and treatments as well as supporting people with dementia, their carers and families. They also support bereaved carers. Being involved with

Rare Dementia Support also enables people to be in contact with others affected by similar conditions.

There are other centres that specialise in dementia research in the UK. These include the Association for Dementia Studies at the University of Worcester; the Dementia Services Development Centre at the University of Stirling and the Centre for Applied Dementia Studies, University of Bradford. These are not NHS facilities but they collaborate with the NHS in researching into different aspects of dementia and developing ways of better supporting people living with dementia and their carers.

## Intermediate care and reablement services

Intermediate care and reablement services are free, short term, time limited services. Their chief aims are to prevent unnecessary hospital admissions and to provide intensive rehabilitation to people who have been discharged from hospital in order to help them return to living as independently as possible and avoid the need for readmission. Intermediate care services can be funded and provided by the NHS or by the local authority. Arrangements vary locally, and can involve the NHS or the local authority individually, or both working together in partnership. Reablement is a form of intermediate care that takes place in the person's own home. As the name suggests it is about restoring confidence and helping people to rediscover and use skills they might have lost. Support staff usually visit the person daily and will observe, guide and encourage them to do things for themselves as much as possible. Intermediate care is time limited (usually six weeks) but if someone still needs care after this time they will need to be assessed for means-tested social care. Most areas also operate a crisis response service to prevent hospital admissions in cases of emergency. This can involve the person being moved on a short term basis to a suitable care home.

Intermediate care services are not specifically for people with dementia, although many people with dementia benefit from them. Some areas operate their own dementia reablement services whose staff are specially trained in dementia and dementia care. A few localities offer an enhanced reablement project, which is led by a psychiatric nurse and provides support to people with complex needs, including memory. Different areas might name their intermediate care services differently but the principles are still the same. Members of the local primary health care team such as a GP or District Nurse can advise about how to access intermediate care.

## NHS continuing healthcare and NHS-funded nursing care

In the UK, the distinction between nursing and social care and how they are funded can be a complex and contentious issue (King's Fund, 2021). The four home countries have different policies on the funding of nursing and social care. For example, in Scotland, people aged 65 and over can receive free personal and nursing care. Whereas for people living in England, Wales and Northern Ireland adult social care is means tested, leaving many people funding a substantial part, if not all, of their own care. Social workers in these three countries need to know about NHS CHC and NHS-FNC (Department of Health and Social Care, 2018b).

NHS CHC is available to adults with long-term, ongoing complex health needs, known as a 'primary health need'. The primary health need concept was introduced in order to help work out whether the local authority or the NHS is responsible for meeting and/or funding a person's care requirements. People who qualify for NHS CHC get their nursing *and* social care funded by the NHS. Unlike social care it is not means tested and covers the costs of someone's health and social care needs. For example, someone resident in a care home who receives NHS CHC can have their care home costs paid for by the NHS. However, NHS CHC can be provided in a variety of settings, including the person's own home.

A diagnosis of dementia does not necessarily mean the someone qualifies for NHS CHC, it depends on how complex and severe the person's needs are. To qualify for NHS CHC, the person needs to be assessed by a team of healthcare professionals. Requesting an assessment can either be done via the GP or by contacting the local clinical commissioning group (CCG) and asking for the NHS CHC coordinator.

---

**BOX 6.1  CONTINUING HEALTHCARE: USEFUL GUIDANCE**

The NHS has produced a helpful video – NHS England Continuing Healthcare (CHC) – that explains the various stages of the process. It is available on YouTube www.youtube.com/watch?v=9xE2oGVRqvY The NHS has also has produced a booklet *NHS continuing healthcare and NHS-FNC* (Department of Health and Social Care, 2018c) which also explains the process.

---

Although social workers do not decide on CHC eligibility they can play an important role in the process by completing the CHC checklist with the person and/or their carers. The CHC checklist is a screening tool to help practitioners identify people who may need a referral for a full assessment of eligibility for NHS CHC.

There is an appeal process if an application for CHC does not prove successful but it can be a long and complex process. Social workers can be useful in assisting people with this. Alternatively, independent advocacy organisations can help or there are private companies that will assist, often on a 'no win no fee' basis. In England, the social enterprise Beacon offers advice and support on all aspects of the CHC process. Independent Health Complaints Advocates can also help with appeals as well as assisting someone with making a complaint about how CHC process has been handled. There is no reliable data on how many appeals are made and how many decisions are overturned (NAO, 2017). However, anecdotal evidence suggests that it is usually worth appealing if an application is turned down.

## NHS-funded nursing care

FNC specifically applies to people who are in a nursing home. If someone has been rejected for NHS CHC funding, but still needs nursing care, they can apply to their local CCG NHS CHC coordinator for NHS-FNC. It will not cover all their care costs but it should cover any care that the person requires from a registered nurse. NHS-FNC is not assessed or means-tested.

In summary:

- NHS CHC covers the full costs of receiving full-time care, whether at home or in a care home, hospice or other care facility. Support is normally reviewed within 3 months and thereafter at least annually. It can be withdrawn following a review.
- FNC is a weekly benefit paid to people who need some nursing care, but who are deemed ineligible for full CHC funding. There must be an assessment for NHS CHC funding first.

## Personal health budgets

From 2014, people in England receiving NHS CHC and Continuing Care have had the 'right to have' a personal health budget. A personal health budget is not additional money, it is a way of giving people the choice in how their agreed care and support plan is put into action. Personal health budgets are the NHS equivalent of personal budgets in local authority social care. Therefore, for example, personal health budgets can be used for employing personal assistants or agency staff, for paying for respite care or assistive technology. A key point is that whatever the budget is spent on has to be agreed by the CCG. If someone with dementia wants to consider this option, they should contact either their GP or the NHS team helping them.

Social workers and health professionals can help the person combine their personal health budget and personal budget to create a personalised and coherent package to meet all their health and social care needs (Community Care, 2019). When working well, personal health budgets can provide more choice and control over the way care and support is delivered for people with dementia. The greater flexibility can also be more beneficial for carers. Personal health budgets can, for example, be a way of ensuring more individually tailored respite care arrangements.

## Activity 6.1: Get to know your local dementia health services

A challenge for anyone with dementia or anyone working with them is navigating around the system of different health services available and understanding the roles of different professionals. Dementia health services are not the same in every area. For example, as discussed, some areas have a dementia advisor service, some have dementia care coordinators and others Admiral nurses. It cannot be taken for granted that these same roles exist in all local areas.

- Make a list of the various primary and secondary health care services that you think are most likely to be needed by people with dementia (and their carers) as the disease progresses.
- Make that sure you know how those services operate and are accessed in your local area.
- Is there a dementia advisor or dementia care coordinator service locally?
- Choose one service and contact them with a view to finding more by, if possible, shadowing a worker, observing sessions, or interviewing staff and service users.
- If someone needed tertiary health care in your area, where would they most likely be referred to?

## Palliative, end of life and hospice services

Chapter 4 explained the principles and policies underpinning palliative and end of life care for people with dementia. Palliative care is focused on effective pain management, symptom control and maintaining the person's dignity and their physical and psychological comfort, particularly as the disease progresses. It is also about supporting families and carers. Chapter 4 also explained about ACP which is how someone with dementia, who still retains capacity, can let it be known what arrangements they would want for their care once they reach a point where they no longer have mental capacity. This can include arrangements for end of life care. The situation can be complicated by the fact that the exact course of any individual's dementia is not easily predictable and preferences might change or no longer be suitable as the disease progresses. This can be very difficult for carers and social workers need to be aware of this and support carers as much as the person through the various fluctuations in the 'end of life' stages. This can be where the concept of ambiguous loss discussed in Chapter 5 is appropriate. As a social work practitioner, support can either be offered personally or by signposting to more specialist support services.

### Palliative care services

The majority of palliative care is provided through the NHS with referrals coming from either the person's GP or another health professional. Sometimes private or charitable service providers take on the role if the person or their family has chosen home-based end-of-life care.

Palliative care is multi-disciplinary and palliative care teams can be hospital or community based. They utilise the facilities and services from a variety of different specialists including palliative care nursing, doctors, psychologists, community teams, social workers, community pharmacies and complementary therapists.

## Hospice services

Hospices are not just for people dying and in the last few weeks or days of their lives. Hospices provide a range of medical and non-medical palliative care services for people with life-limiting conditions. Most hospices are run by charities but with the aid of NHS and local authority funding in many cases. They can either provide palliative care at the hospice or in the community. Care is usually free to the service user. Every nurse, doctor and any other care professional attached to a hospice is a specialist in palliative care but not necessarily in dementia care. Within the hospice movement it is recognised that, whilst hospices are specialists in providing end of life care, some hospices are more advanced than others in the extent to which they are able to fully meet the needs of people with dementia (Hospice UK, 2015). Hospices are now working in closer partnership with dementia care services to improve this.

### Case Study 6.1:   Veronica

Veronica is a 73 year old woman with Alzheimer's that was first diagnosed eight years previously. She is also suffering from terminal bowel cancer. Veronica lives at home and is supported by carers, specialist nursing and her two daughters. Her daughters live nearby and take it in turns to stay in the spare room. Veronica cannot verbalise, but because of the pain she is in, screams frequently and groans loudly. She struggles with transfers unaided and is assessed as being at high risk of falling. This is concerning because the pain and anxiety she is experiencing is making Veronica agitated and she makes frequent efforts to get out of her chair. She also has difficulty eating and swallowing, so needs help with feeding. Because of her pain, anxiety and discomfort Veronica has not slept for several nights which has left her daughters exhausted, very stressed and emotional. With the situation deteriorating and after discussions with Veronica's GP and the Macmillan nurse involved, Donna, the Admiral nurse, referred Veronica to her local hospice In Patient Unit (IPU). This was so that Veronica's symptoms could be controlled and her pain managed better and, importantly, to give the carers and family a break.

On her arrival at the IPU the medical and nursing team carried out a holistic assessment with Veronica and checked with the family whether there were any advance directives. In order to support Veronica with her physical and emotional needs, the unit allocated Healthcare Assistants to carry out an assessment over the first 48 hours after admission. They also completed a behaviour chart for this period, enabling the nursing and medical staff to identify patterns in pain and behavioural issues. All the patients on the unit have a 'what matters to me' form completed with help from family members. This form includes the main issues that are important to Veronica and any other patient/family wishes. Also in discussion with the family the nursing team took note of Veronica's interests in order that she could be suitably engaged and distracted if showing signs of anxiety or agitation. They noted that Veronica enjoyed listening to music on the radio and having the newspaper read to her. Staff were able to assist Veronica with both of these activities. Veronica's routine at home was also included in the assessment and the care staff tried to replicate this as much as practicable. For example, the unit staff made sure that the knitted comfort doll that she used at home was with her whenever she wanted it and that she was able to go outside to the garden in the morning. Any likely changes to routines were discussed with her family.

Due to her Alzheimer's Veronica was unable to express her pain numerically (i.e. on a scale 0–10). Consequently, for the purposes of symptom management and pain control several methods were used including observations of non-verbal signs. Under the supervision of a Palliative Care Consultant the staff used the Pain Assessment in Advanced Dementia Scale (PAINAD). The following areas of assessment were taken into account:

1   Breathing (ranging from normal to laboured and noisy breathing).
2   Negative vocalisation (ranging from being relaxed to repeated troubled calling out and crying).
3   Facial expression (ranging from smiling to facial grimacing).
4   Body language (relaxed to rigid, fists clenching and striking out).
5   Consolability (ranging from no need to console to unable to console).

After observing Veronica for at least five minutes, the scoring system of 1–3 for mild pain; 4–6 for moderate pain and 7–10 for severe pain was used for each of the areas. The PAINAD tool meant that hospice staff could monitor Veronica's pain levels and, consequently, they were able to administer medication and healthcare appropriate to her needs.

During her stay on the unit Veronica was stabilised in terms of comfort and pain control. Staff ensured that not only her physical but her emotional needs were met. Veronica was also able to enjoy listening to music, to spend time in the garden and to have visitors. A volunteer read the newspaper to her. In addition to the medical and nursing interventions, Veronica was also given head, foot and hand massages by the complementary therapy team. This had a noticeably soothing effect. Overall, Veronica was calmer and more settled as a result of the care she received. The stay also provided much needed respite for her family. Now the links have been made with the hospice, Veronica can return to stay when appropriate and benefit from the hospice's Hospice at Home service. Thanks to the work of professionals such as the Admiral and Macmillan nurses, health care assistants, doctors and others much of the stress and anxiety, physical and emotional pain had been taken from this final stage in Veronica's life.

Case Study 6.1 provides an illustration of the ways in which palliative and hospice care can provide comfort to someone with dementia who is in pain and has complex health needs. Hospice services are based on a holistic and person–centred approach. This means that, in addition to medical and nursing interventions, people are enabled to maintain their daily routines as far as possible and they can continue to use their own familiar sources of comfort. Hospices also offer a range of complementary therapies such as aromatherapy and massage which can be very beneficial in promoting physical and mental wellbeing.

## Social care services

Social workers work closely with social care services such as domiciliary, day and residential care, most of which are now provided by the independent sector. Funding arrangements vary across the four nations of the UK. In Scotland, personal and/or nursing care is available to all adults who have been assessed by the local authority as eligible for these services free of charge. In England, Wales and Northern Ireland people eligible for services might be required to pay for their social care depending on a means test. People whose finances take them over the threshold need to fund their own care. When local authorities fund social care, it also normal for them to arrange it. However, people who are assessed as needing to self-fund are often left to find and arrange care themselves, often without the necessary skills to do so (Baxter, Wilberforce and Birks, 2020). In some cases, people who are thought likely to self-fund are screened out of the assessment process altogether. This is despite the fact that the Care Act 2014 in England states that local authorities must carry out an assessment of anyone who appears to require care and support, regardless of their likely eligibility for state-funded care. However, the Act gives people whose savings exceed the means test limits the 'right to request'. Once the request has been made, the authority has a legal duty to meet their eligible needs, even though they will not be entitled to any financial assistance. It is important for social workers to know this because the number of people with dementia who need to fund their own care is rising and they must be given assistance to find the services that will meet their needs. They and their carers should not be left to try to navigate the care system on their own. Some local authorities employ workers whose role is assist self-funders find the appropriate care.

## Personal budgets

As has been highlighted in various places throughout this book, the personalisation agenda requires that social care should be person-centred rather than service led. To this end the introduction of personal budgets has enabled service users to choose or 'co-produce' their own care solutions within an agreed budget. According to the Alzheimer's Society (2016b) local authorities have not always provided either information about or assistance with personal budgets that has been suitable for people with dementia and their carers. The Alzheimer's Society have produced a guide for local authorities *Making personal budgets dementia friendly* (Alzheimer's Society, 2016b). Much of the guide is about the need for local authorities to provide helpful information about how personal budgets work for people with dementia in a user-friendly and timely way. It is also important for potential users of personal budgets to be given information about local organisations whose role is to advise and assist with self-directed support – specifically Direct Payments. Without the help of these specialist organisations, many people would not be able to use a Direct Payment to employ a personal assistant.

## The state of social care

In 2009, Anthea Innes wrote the following about the gap between the 'theory' and practice of dementia care:

> Care ideals may remain viewed as a utopian vision if, at the ground level, such ideals are not translated into tangible and concrete examples of how to provide the type of care that those writing about care practices, such as policy makers and academics, advocate. Those working at the coalface of service delivery are often not given adequate resources, support and training to enable them to put into place the ideals set from those who are at least one step removed from the reality of providing care. Thus, ideals may not even be known by those delivering care, with training opportunities limited to staff higher up the care-delivery hierarchy and information-sharing mechanisms which offer recommendations about care delivery confined to written reports that are not widely read by care practitioners.
>
> *(Innes, 2009: 12)*

Unfortunately, at the time of writing, over a decade later, little has changed, particularly in respect of the system of social care in the UK. In addition to the issues highlighted by Innes, the sector continues to experience workforce problems with low pay, high staff turnover and inadequate training which have still not been fully addressed. The consequences for people with dementia who use social care services is that their needs are not always well met. As members of the social care work-force, there is a role to play for social workers in both campaigning from within the system for improvements and encouraging others, in and outside of the system, to fight for change, including better funding and better training for the workforce.

## Domiciliary care

The care needs of people with dementia change over time. For many, their first experience of social care is a domiciliary service and, for some, that is the only social care service that they will use. Most domiciliary care is provided by privately run care agencies. The care tasks they undertake tend to mainly involve personal care such as getting people up from bed, washing, dressing and providing food. High turnover of staff in the care sector means that agencies can often send a variety of different carers to the same person (Skills for Care, 2020). When this happens it can be confusing for the person, it can disrupt continuity of care and prevent a trusting care relationship from forming. Without being overly alarmist and pessimistic, social workers can help prepare service users for the possibility of this happening when they are discussing care options. Care agencies also vary in the extent to which they have expertise in caring for people with dementia. Social workers can either carry out their own checks via the CQC online portal to see if a particular agency has dementia specialist care trained staff. For example, it is possible for agencies to achieve Dementia Champion accredited provider status. Alternatively, they can advise people and their carers how to do this for themselves. It is important that people can make informed decisions and have choices.

## Day care

'Day care' is an umbrella term can refer to any care arrangement that takes place during the day outside of the person's own home. Day care usually takes place in some form of designated day centre, but need not do. It could be in a church hall, community centre, a private establishment or some other location. Day centres are mainly run by independent sector organisations. Day centres *per se* are not subject to registration or inspection by the CQC. Some centres are attached to care homes but others can be in different locations. Mostly, day centres charge an attendance fee. Some day centres provide their own transport but others do not. Service users need to make their own arrangements which, for some, might involve the use of a voluntary driver scheme. Transport arrangements to day care and associated costs need to be clarified at the outset with potential service users.

Not all providers of day care have specialist dementia trained staff and they might not be particularly 'dementia friendly'. However, the needs of people with dementia vary considerably, so potential users should be informed of all their day care options whether the provider has a dementia specialism or not. With someone whose needs are more complex and whose dementia has advanced it is important that the day centre is fully dementia friendly, with staff properly qualified and trained. Specialist dementia day centres will be able to set up appropriate activities and will have appropriate safety measures in place. Whatever the choice of day care arrangement, good practice is to arrange a trial visit for a morning or afternoon so that all parties involved can make an assessment of suitability. Sometimes when somebody is referred to day care, a member of staff from the centre will visit the person in their home to make an assessment. This is good practice because it allows the day centre to get a better sense of the person by seeing them in their home context.

Apart from providing the person with dementia with social, creative and other therapeutic opportunities, day care provides a break in daily care for the person's family carers. Giving family carers support and respite by using day care can have a positive impact on the relationship between them and the person with dementia (Maffioletti et al., 2019). That said, someone with dementia should not be coerced into a day care arrangement purely to provide the carers with respite, even if it is much needed. There must be some tangible benefit for the person with dementia.

### Activity 6.2: Get to know your local dementia day care services

1   Find out what day care provision is available for people at different stages of dementia.
2   How well does provision cater for diversity in terms of age, gender, ethnicity, disability and in other ways?
3   How well does provision cater for people with complex health needs?
4   Is the provision dementia friendly? Give reasons.
5   Do staff have specialist dementia training?
6   What are the costs and transport arrangements?
7   Arrange to visit a centre that caters specifically for people with dementia. What sort of experiences and care does it offer? What is your assessment? Would you be happy for a relative of yours to attend if they were living with dementia?

### *Care homes*

There are two main types of care home – residential care homes and nursing homes. What differentiates a residential care home from a nursing home is that, as part of their registration, nursing homes must have a qualified nurse on site. This means they can offer a higher level of care, especially for people with complex needs. In general, nursing home care costs more for this reason. In the UK, although local authorities still run some care homes, most are now privately owned or run by charities and voluntary organisations such as Abbeyfield. The majority of the people living in care homes in the UK actually have some form of dementia. However, people with dementia in residential and care homes might be cared for alongside people living with other long-term and complex health needs such as Parkinson's Disease, diabetes or lung disease. Often care homes will have a reference to 'dementia' on their website, this does not mean that the home is a specialist in dementia care but that, amongst their residents, they have people with dementia. It is always best to arrange a visit, speak to a manager and spend some time in the home before deciding about it. A manager should be able to answer questions about how many carers have been trained in dementia care and what level of qualification they have. A visit also provides a good opportunity to get a sense of the home's ambience, amenities, state of repair and care culture. Family carers often ask social workers for recommendation about care homes. Social workers should be wary about doing this as it is not their really their role. The most appropriate response is to give carers the information to make their own choice – together with the person with dementia if they have the capacity. However, generally speaking, social workers should not really discuss a care home with a family without having visited it themselves.

In some areas, there are 'dementia care centres' which specialise in providing dementia care only. They are usually, but not always, registered as nursing homes. These specialist dementia care homes are designed to provide an appropriate caring environment for people with dementia. This might be, for example, by using simple, clear signage and specific colours on doors, carpets and corridors enable residents to recognise where they are and to find their way around. There are often other features such as sensory gardens, designed to stimulate the senses through touch, sight, taste and hearing. As 'sundowning' can be a common occurrence in people living with dementia, the environment can be designed to calm agitation and lighting used to help residents understand what time it is and whether it is day or night. Areas where residents can engage in supervised gardening are sometimes provided. The principles upon which dementia care centres are based means that they should be able to deliver person-centred dementia care, including life story work, creative activities and other therapeutic interventions. However, the extent to which these activities take place varies – often to do with the availability of activities coordinators and other specialists. Again, the choice of a dementia care centre needs to be made on at least one visit to assess the care culture and the facilities it has available.

Dementia care homes are usually designed with safety as a major priority. So, whilst there is often free access for residents to move around the rooms inside the building and to any gardens, external doors to the street are locked. Article 5 of the Human Rights Act 1998 states that 'everyone has the right to liberty and security of person. No one shall be deprived of his or her liberty [unless] in accordance with a procedure prescribed in law'. As a consequence, England, Wales, Scotland and Northern Ireland all have legal safeguards in place to protect people's rights to liberty in care homes. Therefore, to lock doors to prevent a resident from leaving, the care home must follow the procedures laid down in relevant legislation. At the time of writing for England and Wales these are the DoLs procedures as specified in the Mental Capacity Act 2005. DoLs are due to be replaced by Liberty Protection

Safeguards (LPS) sometime in 2022. The important point is that the use of locked doors in dementia care settings always need to be justified, with the proper procedures and legal guidelines having been followed.

Moving someone with dementia to a care home is more often a decision taken by family carers rather than by the person themselves. However, when social workers become involved it is important that the perspective of the person is given the fullest possible consideration. It is also very important that the care and support plan put together by the social worker contains as much information as possible about who they are, their needs, and preferences. The care and support plan should focus on the person's specific care needs and their physical and mental health needs. It should contain information about how to manage their pain, control their anxiety, and manage sleep disturbances and agitated behaviour. However, it is equally important to use the care and support plan bring the person to life as an individual. So, for example, it should explain how the person likes to be called, who and what is meaningful to them in their lives, what their occupation was, what their hobbies were, what they like doing now and so on. The care home will formulate their own care plans but it is very useful for them to have the social work care and support plan for reference.

Well run care homes should arrange for a senior member of staff to visit the person at home, or in hospital, and, if possible invite them or their family carers to view the care home before agreeing that they can meet their needs. Preparation is key to ensure a smooth transition in what is a critical moment in the person's life (Fossey, 2014). If a member of the care home staff has assessed the person in their own home, ideally they should be there to welcome them to the home when the move takes place.

It is not inevitable that people with dementia will need to go and live in a care home. However, it is probably something that is on the mind of most people with dementia and their family caregivers at various points, even if they choose to reject it as an option. It is also a choice that can be rejected and reconsidered as the person's health deteriorates. It is not uncommon for people with dementia to be discharged into a care home from hospital having experienced a significant deterioration in their health. Partly to ease pressure on beds, sometimes these decisions are presented to the person and their family as a *fait accompli*. However, they need not and should not be. Moving into a care home is always an important, complex and consequential decision. Social workers must ensure that the person's best interests are promoted, that a proper assessment is made, a detailed care and support plan put together and that genuine choices are offered to the person and their family. If the decision is to transfer to a care home the best possible preparation should be undertaken. Failure to do any of these things will mean that the person's quality of life and wellbeing risks being severely diminished at a critical stage in their life. The pressure to move people out of hospital is known to be a source of tension between medical, nursing and social work staff and it can be hard for hospital social workers, in particular, to resist the power of the doctors and nurses (Heenan, 2021). It is, however, an important part of the social work role to safeguard the rights of vulnerable adults and to promote their best interests. A hasty and rushed discharge to an alien environment for anyone, let alone someone with dementia, is definitely not in their best interests.

## Therapeutic activities

Creative activities such as dancing, singing and art can be very therapeutic for people living with dementia. Although some are available formally as 'Art Therapy' or 'Music Therapy' via the NHS or other health and social care organisations, beneficial creative activities are often provided by local voluntary groups. Consequently, the availability of these types of activity varies from one area to another. Funding is a critical factor and most voluntary groups would expect a small fee from participants to cover costs.

### *Art and crafts*

Engagement with art and the arts in their broadest sense can provide meaning, purpose and value to people living with dementia (Basting, 2014; Craig, 2004). The benefits of either observing art or engaging in painting, drawing or various other craft and making activities (even doing jigsaws) are many and diverse. They help promote wellbeing and aid self-expression. Being part of an art group brings enjoyment, enables people to be 'in the moment', to be creative and to make social connections. Arts sessions can also provide opportunities for the person to exercise skills in choice and in the expression of preferences and feelings. However, this raises questions of how the group is run and the degree to which the people attending it are in control of the group's activities (Craig, 2004). Some people prefer a well-structured, tutor-led session but others like to be able to exercise a large degree of choice in what they do. So matching the person to the group is important. If the right opportunities can be found then it is very likely that the person's mental wellbeing will be boosted significantly. If nothing else, involving oneself in art and craft activities can provide a distraction from anxiety and rumination about one's poor health.

### *Music and singing groups*

There is a large and growing body of evidence that shows that participation in different musical activities has a range of benefits for people with mental ill health including those living with dementia. Musical activity provides opportunities for self-expression, boosts self-esteem and helps maintain both mental and physiological wellbeing (Richards, 2020; Bowell and Bamford, 2018). Musical activities also facilitate social contact when done collectively. Critically, Richards (2020) states that 'music is especially beneficial in dementia care as, whilst other cognitive abilities deteriorate, musical memory remains intact (p. 19).' Music can be used in different ways, including:

- helping to prompt memories;
- helping to form a connection to others;

- accompanying reminiscence and life story work;
- creating a calming environment;
- creating a convivial environment;
- as an accompaniment to dancing and other physical activities;
- providing opportunities for singing, which has its own health and mood enhancing benefits. Singing is also good for lung health.

Music can also provide opportunities for family carers to reconnect with the person in ways which are positive, energizing and enjoyable, partly because they are not specifically to do with the caring role.

The Memory Notes group in Cambridge have made a short film available on You-Tube 'Memory Notes The Movie' (www.youtube.com/watch?v=V17lRyCH2nU) which illustrates many of the benefits for people with dementia and their carers of singing as part of a group.

In the spirit of holistic and person-centred practice, social workers need to ensure that they are aware of the range of therapeutic groups and creative activities available to people with dementia and their carers in their local area. They are not always easy to locate. A recent report (Bowell and Bamford, 2018) observed that 'the dementia and music environment is supported by a dedicated network of individuals and organisations' (p. 7) but they added that such provision in the UK is sporadic in its coverage and underfunded.

Whilst it is not usually the case that social workers need to refer people to these services and groups in any formal sense, they can help people make a choice by finding out appropriate information and signposting them. In the UK, the organisation *Arts 4 Dementia* (arts4dementia.org.uk) is a useful source of information on the different types of artistic groups running in different localities. Social workers in the UK should also aim to discover whether there is a NHS Social Prescribing Link worker in their area. This is a role that has been created in order to support people with complex, long-term and mental health conditions by linking them to community groups. These groups can sometimes involve the sort of activities discussed here, although they might not specifically be for people with dementia.

## Technology enabled care (telecare, telehealth, assistive, monitoring, surveillance and carer support technologies)

The term 'technology enabled care' is used to describe the range of technology that enables people with disabilities and health conditions to live independently and safely. The technology can take many forms (CQC, 2020b). The increased use of technology as a means of delivering improved and more personalised health and social care services has been signalled in national policies for some time (e.g. Department of Health, 2005b). According to World Health Organisation (2004: 10) 'assistive technology' is defined as an 'umbrella term for any device or system that allows individuals to perform tasks they would otherwise be unable to do or increases the ease and safety with which tasks can be performed'. Coming under this umbrella term are low tech solutions such as ramps, rails, chair risers and perching stools and increasingly high tech solutions such as hearing aids, electric wheel chairs, screen magnifiers, fall sensor alarm systems and voice recognition devices. Over the years, more and more sophisticated technology has been invented to meet the needs of people with different types of impairments whether this be: mobility problems, sensory impairments, cognitive problems or combinations of these.

Telecare and telehealth also fall under the umbrella of technology enabled care. Telecare uses technologies such as remote monitoring and emergency alarms to enable people to receive care at home and live as independently as possible. An example would be where the person wears a pendant which has a button they can press if they fall or require assistance for some other reason. The button will alert a care agency who will call back and either send someone to investigate or alert a nominated carer. Alternatively, there are fall detectors that will automatically alert the care agency if the person falls and is unable to press the button. Other types of remote sensor are also available.

Despite the fact that telecare has now been in existence for many years, the current evidence base does not provide conclusive confirmation of its appropriateness or efficacy for people with dementia (Lariviere et al., 2021). It needs to be seen as a complement to rather than a substitute for proper person-centred care. It also needs to be used in a way that demonstrably benefits the person with dementia rather than just providing caregivers with 'peace of mind', important as that is. That said, there are a range of options now available and, if used appropriately, they can be used to improve the lives of both the person with dementia and their family and carers. The Alzheimer's Society (2019) has produced a useful factsheet '*Using technology to help with everyday life*' that provides information about the range of technology available, the costs and how to obtain it. It also provides guidance on how to decide what technology to get and how to use it. As the leaflet says 'the technology should work for you, and not the other way around' (p. 3).

Telecare services, like most assistive technology, can be bought and arranged privately or can be accessed by contacting an NHS or local authority Occupational Therapist who will make their assessment and will be able to advise what is the most appropriate form of technology to use. GPs and other primary health care workers should be able to supply the contact details of the local Occupational Therapy team.

The assistive technology appropriate for someone with dementia obviously depends on their individual situation and their particular needs. In addition to those discussed, there are technologies that can help people who have developed various types of cognitive impairment. These include door sensors that will let another person know if the person with dementia leaves their home and might need help; bed sensors that will raise an alarm if someone gets out of bed; door sensors that raise an alarm if a door is opened and heat detectors which will set off an alarm if the temperature in the kitchen is very high, which might indicate that something is burning. In addition, there are medication dispensers which can be programmed to open and dispense the correct dosage of medication only when it should be taken.

In addition to the monitoring devices described, some families are now installing CCTV cameras in the homes of relatives with dementia in order to monitor their behaviour and, in some cases, the behaviour of carers. Sometimes this is done covertly and without the knowledge or consent of the person with dementia. The expansion of remote monitoring and surveillance technology in care generally, but dementia care specifically, raises important ethical and legal issues, not least about the privacy, rights and restrictions on the liberty of the person being monitored, but also about the storage of any recorded data and who has access to it. In addition to these issues, there is the risk that being made a subject of surveillance technologies, for whatever reason, can contribute towards stigmatisation – including self-stigmatisation (Vermeer, Higgs and Charlesworth, 2019). The principles of rights-based and person-centred dementia care means that the installation of any form of technology definitely needs to be in the 'best interests' of the person with dementia. Legally, it could be said that any such installation is a breach of the Article 8 of the Human Rights Act 1998 which asserts the right to a private life. However, essentially, it is a legal grey area so any decisions to install CCTV need to be weighed carefully (CQC, 2015). The person's safety and the 'peace of mind' of carers are important factors to take into consideration but they should be balanced in such a way that leaves the person with dementia not just safe but with the best quality of life possible, which means taking their privacy and dignity into account.

Telehealth is a system to monitor someone's health remotely via telecommunications technology. This can be by using text messages, automated phone calls or apps to help people manage their own health condition. It is important to note that telehealth requires a reliable broadband connection. Details about what telehealth technologies are available locally should be available via the GP or local primary health care team.

With the use of any type of technology enabled care it is important that the informed consent of the person is sought. If they do not have the mental capacity to consent, a 'best interests' decision would need to be made within the provisions of the Mental Capacity Act 2005 and associated codes and practice guidance.

Finally, health and social care professionals and carers need to guard against the unintended consequences of using assistive technology. For example, the use of software like Zoom proved valuable during the Covid-19 pandemic to enable families to keep in touch during Government imposed lockdowns. However, if remote, online communication becomes the default, with no attempt to incorporate face to face contact, this risks seriously impoverishing the life and wellbeing of the person with dementia. There is also the risk, in some cases, that any type of remote technology might create anxiety or even a level of paranoia in the person with dementia. This suggests that the use of technology enabled care, in its many forms, should always be closely monitored, with the perspective of the person using it always taken into account and adjustments made accordingly.

# Advocacy services

## Statutory independent advocacy

As outlined in Chapter 3, people living with dementia might qualify for the services of an independent advocate in ensuring that their voice and participation is facilitated in key decision making processes concerning their health, housing and social care. The Care Act 2014, Mental Capacity Act 2005 and Mental Health 2007 set out the precise conditions that must be met for an independent advocate to be offered in England. Independent advocacy is available under different legislation in the other UK nations but the role is more or less the same. It is important that social workers make service users aware of their rights to independent advocacy and also let them and their carers know how to access it. Most local authorities commission independent advocacy from national organisations such as VoiceAbility, POhWER and SEAP but this varies across the UK. The Scottish Independent Advocacy Alliance promotes and supports independent advocacy services across Scotland and their website offers an online database of advocacy services. Organisations that provide statutory independent advocacy should be able to offer non-instructed advocacy for people with dementia who no longer have the mental capacity to express their preferences, wishes and feelings (Scourfield, 2021). To uphold the rights of people with dementia it is important for social workers to know about the role of statutory independent advocates and how they can be accessed.

## Other advocacy organisations

Outside of these statutory roles there are other forms of advocacy and other organisations that can help represent the interests of people with dementia. This is not just in relation to the health and social care system but also with other matters, for example, housing or welfare rights issues. There are many national and local voluntary organisations who provide advocacy as part of their service provision. This is not necessarily statutory advocacy such as that defined by the Care, Mental Health or Mental Capacity Acts. It might be more broadly described as community advocacy. This form of advocacy is not necessarily targeted at people with dementia but might be offered to people who come into certain group categories. For example, AGE UK offers advice and advocacy services to older people and MIND offers advocacy services to people with mental health problems. More specifically for people with dementia, the Alzheimer's Society and the Dementia Action Alliance campaign for people with dementia nationally and can also signpost to local organisations.

Advocacy is an important part of the social work role, and social workers should see themselves as advocates for their service users with dementia. However, at times, social workers can be conflicted in how far they can take the side of the service user by their responsibilities to their employing organisation and the fact that of being part of the health and social care system (Scourfield, 2021). Therefore, it is good for people with dementia to be able to have a choice of advocate service and for social workers to be able to offer that choice.

## Self-advocacy

It would be stereotyping people living with dementia to believe that they always need someone else to advocate for them. It is important for people with dementia to be able to self-advocate as far as possible – both as individuals and collectively. The ability to self-advocate effectively is empowering for the individual. However, more generally, people with dementia speaking up for themselves also helps to counter the stigma and negative attitudes towards dementia described in earlier chapters, that is to say, dementia-ism. Dementia Alliance International, the Alzheimer's Society UK and the 3 Nations Dementia Working Group have collaborated to produce a Directory of Resources specifically to support dementia self-advocates (Dementia Alliance International, 2019). Dementia Alliance International describes itself as 'a collaboration of like-minded individuals diagnosed with dementia providing a unified voice of strength, advocacy, and support in the fight for individual autonomy for people with dementia' (www.dementiaallianceinternational.org/about-dai/). Membership of Dementia Alliance International is free and is open to anyone with a diagnosis of any type of dementia.

The rationale for self-advocacy is well put by Kate Swaffer, who was diagnosed with young onset dementia. In the video 'The Many Voices of Dementia' produced by Dementia Alliance International (www.youtube.com/watch?v=5eeepLmDQAI), Swaffer says, 'Why did I become a self-advocate for dementia? Because I got sick of people without dementia telling me how I felt and what was best for me'.

Self-advocacy is not a 'service' as such but social workers could introduce people with dementia with whom they are working to organisations such as Dementia Alliance International and Dementia Action Alliance as a possible method of empowerment.

## Dementia friends

Dementia Friends (www.dementiafriends.org.uk) is an initiative set up by the Alzheimer's Society. It is an advocacy organisation in the sense that it is a campaign to change people's perceptions of dementia and to transform the way society thinks, acts and talks about dementia. Its aim is to make communities more 'dementia friendly'. Much of the work is about raising awareness, countering stereotypes, providing education, information and humanising narratives and promoting social inclusion. As well as encouraging individuals to become Dementia Friends Champions, organisations are encouraged to get involved with the campaign. This is to ensure that work places, private organisations and public bodies are aware of the needs of people living with dementia and are motivated to adapt to meet them as far as possible. Social workers practising in the area of dementia care should consider becoming a Dementia Friend or, at least, find out more about what the initiative is trying to achieve.

## Support organisations

There are different support groups and support organisations for people with different types of dementia, most of which are run with input from people with dementia. The biggest and best known in the UK is the Alzheimer's Society which, despite its name, does not limit its support and advice to people with Alzheimer's. However, there is also Dementia UK (now merged with YoungDementia UK), Alzheimer Scotland in Scotland, Dementia NI in Northern Ireland and Alzheimer's Society Cymru in Wales. There are organisations which are set up to support people living specific types of dementia such as The Lewy Body Society (www.lewybody.org) and Rare Dementia Support (www.raredementiasupport.org). It is worth checking locally what is available because many different groups operate in different localities. Living with dementia can be an isolating and lonely experience. The Alzheimer's Society (www.alzheimers.org.uk/get-support/your-support-services/befriending-people-dementia) can put people in touch with dementia befriending schemes. However, organisations such as AGE UK also operate befriending schemes for people with dementia in some areas, so it is worth doing research locally.

### *Dementia (Memory) Cafés*

Dementia Cafés (sometimes called Memory Cafés) were first developed in the Netherlands The first Dementia café was established in 2000 in the UK and since then many more have been set up These are usually set up by local branches of the Alzheimer's Society, Rotary Clubs or other local charities and voluntary organisations. They are mainly staffed by volunteers. They are designed for people with dementia and their carers, to meet with others in the same situation, to have a cup of tea, chat and share their experiences in a friendly environment. Some Dementia cafés put on social activities, often aimed at improving memory. Although Dementia cafés are praised in many quarters, there is currently not a strong evidence base to confirm their efficacy. However, one study found that:

> One very important finding here is how [Dementia] cafés may help to normalise dementia. They are a safe place where carers and people living with dementia can be themselves and can talk freely about any challenges they might be facing with café providers and other carers. Importantly cafés also give carers an opportunity to observe people living with dementia at varying points in the illness. This can help them feel more confident about the future and reassure them about any future challenges. Importantly, by attending the café, they learn about where they might access other types of support both from services and from other carers.
>
> *(Greenwood et al., 2017: 7)*

The US based website Memory Café Directory (www.memorycafedirectory.com/) maintains a directory of cafés in different countries including the UK. Cafés can also be located via the Alzheimer's Society.

## Support for carers

Most of the national and local dementia support organisations will also provide support to carers. However, there are more carer focused organisations. Carers UK and Carers Trust are well known national organisations but many different local care support groups exist. Some are user-led self-help groups. Dementia Carers Count (dementiacarers.org.uk) not only provides support they also provide courses for carers to help carers understand and cope with living with someone with dementia.

Although, there are many and diverse support groups nationally and locally about which people with dementia and carers can be given the information it has to be recognised that membership of such groups is not for everyone. For some people, they do not want to identify too strongly with the world of dementia and dementia organisations, and this should be respected. They are not necessarily 'in denial', it can be out of the desire to preserve a sense of their personal identity. Others dip in and out of various support activities but without committing themselves to membership, whilst others work out their own support networks and resources. However, even though the people with whom they are working might not need or want to use certain services, social workers should have up-to-date knowledge about what is available so they can offer it.

## Identifying gaps and barriers and contributing to the development of services

A key part of the social work role with people living with dementia involves arranging, matching, referring and signposting them and their carers to different services. The personalisation agenda, as well as the desire for person-centred dementia care, makes providing choice of service a central principle.

In reality, there are several obstacles to providing services that are completely person-centred. However, it is also a key social work role to promote social justice and to contribute to the development of services that are both socially inclusive and culturally sensitive (BASW, 2018). This means that when there are gaps in appropriate services, for whatever reason, this information should be fed through to senior management and service commissioners.

There are particular gaps in appropriate service provision in many rural areas and for minority ethnic groups in some areas (Innes, Archibald and Murphy, 2004; All-Party Parliamentary Group on Dementia, 2013; Mukadam, Cooper and Livingston, 2013). Another long-standing problem is that many dementia services are aimed at older people, which leaves younger people with dementia fewer choices of services that are appropriate to their age (Mayrhofer et al., 2018). The task is not always about stimulating provision where there are gaps. It is also about raising awareness amongst minority groups, promoting the prevention agenda, counteracting stigma and encouraging contact with medical and health services. Much of the work is about being sensitive to how different cultural groups understand mental illness and approach matters of death and dying. Having a more culturally nuanced understanding of why people cannot or do not take up services can help produce more culturally tailored interventions. This has proved to be effective, for example, with South Asian communities (Mukadam, Cooper and Livingston, 2013) and Gypsy and Traveller communities (Lane et al., 2021). Putting marginalised groups in contact with services requires a level of sensitive outreach from suitably qualified workers (Goodorally, 2015). That said, there is a limit to what individual social workers can achieve in this respect. It needs a whole systems approach to bring about the necessary changes. However, social workers can demonstrate professional leadership by drawing attention to where minority groups' needs are not being met and advocating for change.

## An international perspective

Dementia services are developing all the time. Chapter 3 explained how dementia has been put on the policy agenda in the UK in recent years and most of this book has taken the UK, mainly English, perspective. However, dementia is a global issue and it is always useful to take an international perspective for what can be learned from other countries. Japan, for example, has pioneered dementia-friendly communities and has taken steps to change not only thinking about dementia but the language used to describe it to further help the process of destigmatisation. Elsewhere, European countries such as Belgium and Netherlands have been ahead of the UK in their efforts to develop dementia-friendly communities. The Hogeweyk Dementia Village in the Netherlands is one particular innovation attracting attention from around the world as a model to provide an adapted but 'normalised' life for people living with dementia where they can feel both safe and valued (Baumann, 2021).

A global study of dementia-friendly communities and dementia-friendly services found that they are most likely to be successful when people feel valued and safe, when there is an understanding of dementia in the community, when there is continued access, when they are adequately resourced and, critically, when there is input from people with dementia in their design. However, an ongoing challenge is how to involve marginalised and minority groups in this process (Shannon, Bail and Neville, 2019). The overall message from looking at services around the world is that it is beneficial to have a diverse range of services but that this, in isolation, is not enough. The wider society and communities in which the services are delivered must be more inclusive and understanding about dementia. Only then will people with the disease be able to feel that they are being treated with the dignity and respect they deserve as human beings. In the UK and internationally, the goal is to be able to provide a range of dementia-friendly services within a broader social and cultural context that is also dementia-friendly. Services that, in themselves, contribute to the segregation, and marginalisation of people living with dementia might serve some expedient function but are actually part of the problem that people with dementia face – stigmatisation.

## Conclusion

Dementia services are developing all the time. Therefore, this chapter cannot claim to be comprehensive in any way. However, it has discussed a range of services that can benefit people living with dementia and their carers in different ways. Which particular services are most appropriate depends on the person's individual situation, the stage of their dementia and their individual preferences and circumstances. What suits one person might not suit another. However, social workers need to be able to bring to people's attention all the possible alternatives available. It should be reiterated that the whole range of services might not be available in every locality. Another point to highlight is that services that benefit people with dementia need not be medical nor formal health services as such. The chapter has discussed how creative activities, complementary therapies, Dementia cafés and different types of technology-enabled care can promote wellbeing, social inclusion and independence as well as help to provide a safe environment for people in various stages of dementia. The section on advocacy highlighted that, unfortunately, people with dementia still face stigma and marginalisation and that ways of overcoming this need to be explored. Different forms of advocacy, including self-advocacy, are useful tools for empowerment in this respect. Social workers must also become advocates for people with dementia to ensure that their rights to services and their rights as human beings are respected. To end, it should be restated (to paraphrase George Bernard Shaw) that perhaps the greatest social service that can be rendered to someone living with dementia is that, as Tom Kitwood (1997) said, they be treated as a PERSON-with-dementia rather than a person-with-DEMENTIA (p. 7).

## Further reading

Different services are being developed all the time in the UK. Also, unfortunately, some services are cut for various reasons. Therefore, the best way to keep up to date with service provision is by doing research online. The NHS and Alzheimer's Society websites have many useful links. Local authorities also provide a lot of useful information.

Alzheimer's Disease International (2016). *Dementia Friendly Communities Global Developments* (2nd edition). London: Alzheimer's Disease International.
    This report provides a stimulating overview of various developments around the world which aim to produce more dementia-friendly, non-stigmatising and inclusive services.

# REFERENCES

Adams, T. and Bartlett, R. (2003). Constructing dementia. In Adams, T. and Manthorpe, J. (Eds). *Dementia Care*. London: Arnold. 3–21.

Adams, T. and Manthorpe, J. (2003). *Dementia Care*. London: Arnold.

Adelman, S., Blanchard, M. and Livingston, G. (2009). A systematic review of the prevalence and covariates of dementia or relative cognitive impairment in the older African-Caribbean population in Britain. *International Journal of Geriatric Psychiatry*. 24, 657–665.

Age UK (n.d.). *Understanding Dementia*. Retrieved from: www.ageuk.org.uk/information-advice/health-wellbeing/conditions-illnesses/dementia/understanding-dementia/.

Age UK (2021). *Timothy West and Prunella Scales on Dementia*. Retrieved from: www.ageuk.org.uk/information-advice/health-wellbeing/conditions-illnesses/dementia/timothy-west-and-prunella-scales-on-dementia/.

All-Party Parliamentary Group on Dementia (2008). *Always a Last Resort Inquiry into the Prescription of Antipsychotic Drugs to People with Dementia Living in Care Homes*. London: The House of Commons All-Party Parliamentary Group on Dementia.

All-Party Parliamentary Group on Dementia (APPG) (2013). *Dementia Does Not Discriminate. The Experiences of Black, Asian and Minority Ethnic Communities*. London: The House of Commons All-Party Parliamentary Group on Dementia.

All-Party Parliamentary Group on Dementia (APPG) (2019). *Hidden No More: Dementia and Disability*. London: The House of Commons All-Party Parliamentary Group on Dementia.

Allen, K. (2001). *Communication and Consultation: Exploring Ways for Staff to Involve People with Dementia in Developing Services*. Bristol: Policy Press.

Alzheimer's Association (2021). *Down Syndrome and Alzheimer's Disease*. Retrieved from: www.alz.org/alzheimers-dementia/what-is-dementia/types-of-dementia/down-syndrome.

Alzheimer's Disease International (2016). *Dementia Friendly Communities Global Developments* (2nd edition). London: Alzheimer's Disease International.

Alzheimer's Disease International (2019). *World Alzheimer Report 2019 Attitudes to Dementia*. London: Alzheimer's Disease International.

Alzheimer's Research UK (2015). *Women and Dementia a Marginalised Majority*. Cambridge: Alzheimer's Research UK.

Alzheimer's Society (n.d.). *How Do Drugs for Alzheimer's Disease Work?* Retrieved from: www.alzheimers.org.uk/about-dementia/treatments/drugs/how-do-drugs-alzheimers-disease-work.

Alzheimer's Society (2013). *The Dementia Guide: Living Well After Diagnosis.* London: Alzheimer's Society.

Alzheimer's Society (2014). *Drug Treatments for Alzheimer's Disease.* London: Alzheimer's Society.

Alzheimer's Society (2015). *Alzheimer's Society's View on Mistreatment and Abuse of People with Dementia.* Retrieved from: www.alzheimers.org.uk/about-us/policy-and-influencing/what-we-think/mistreatment-and-abuse-people-dementia.

Alzheimer's Society (2016a). *Genetics of Dementia.* London: Alzheimer's Society.

Alzheimer's Society (2016b). *Making Personal Budgets Dementia Friendly a Guide for Local Authorities.* London: Alzheimer's Society.

Alzheimer's Society (2017). *The Dementia Guide: Living Well After Diagnosis.* London: Alzheimer's Society.

Alzheimer's Society (2019). *Using Technology to Help with Everyday Life.* Factsheet 437LP April 2019. London: Alzheimer's Society.

Alzheimer's Society (2021a). *The Progression and Stages of Alzheimer's.* Retrieved from: www.alzheimers.org.uk/about-dementia/symptoms-and-diagnosis/how-dementia-progresses/progression-stages-dementia.

Alzheimer's Society (2021b). *What Is Mixed Dementia?* Retrieved from: www.alzheimers.org.uk/blog/what-is-mixed-dementia#:~:text=Mixed%20dementia%20is%20much%20more,diagnosed%20with%20'mixed%20dementia.

Alzheimer's Society (2021c). *Dementia Tax.* Retrieved from: www.alzheimers.org.uk/about-us/policy-and-influencing/what-we-think/dementia-tax.

Alzheimer's Society (2021d). *End of Life Care.* Retrieved from: www.alzheimers.org.uk/get-support/help-dementia-care/end-life-care.

Aquilina, C. and Hughes, J. (2006). The return of the living dead: Agency lost and found? In Hughes, J., Louw, S. and Sabat, S. (Eds). *Dementia: Mind Meaning and the Person.* Oxford: Oxford University Press. 143–161.

Archibald, C. (2004). Sexuality and Dementia. Beyond the Pale? In Innes, A., Archibald, C. and Murphy, C. (Eds). *Dementia and Social Inclusion.* London: Jessica Kingsley Publishers. 96–112.

Arevalo-Rodriguez, I., Smailagic, N., Roqué I Figuls, M., Ciapponi, A., Sanchez-Perez, E., Giannakou, A., Pedraza, O., Bonfill Cosp, X. and Cullum, S. (2015). Mini-mental state examination (MMSE) for the detection of Alzheimer's disease and other dementias in people with mild cognitive impairment (MCI). *Cochrane Database of Systematic Reviews.* March 5; 2015(3).

Association of Palliative Care Social Workers (2016). *The Role of Social Workers in Palliative, End of Life and Bereavement Care.* Retrieved from: www.apcsw.org.uk/resources/social-work-role-eol.pdf.

Audit Commission (2000). *Forget Me Not.* London: The Stationery Office.

Audit Commission (2002). *Forget Me Not* 2002. London: The Stationery Office.

Banovic, S., Zunic, L. and Sinanovic, O. (2018). Communication difficulties as a result of dementia. *Materia Socio-Medica.* 30(3), 221–224. https://doi.org/10.5455/msm.2018.30.221-224.

Bartlett, R. (2014). The emergent modes of dementia activism. *Ageing & Society.* 34, 623–644.

Basting, A. (2014). The arts in dementia care. In Downs, M. and Bowers, B. (Eds). *Excellence in Dementia Care. Research into Practice* (2nd edition). Maidenhead: Open University Press. 132–143.

BASW (2018). *The Professional Capabilities Framework (PCF)*. Retrieved from: www.basw.co.uk/professional-development/professional-capabilities-framework-pcf/the-pcf.

BASW (2021). *The BASW Code of Ethics for Social Work*. Birmingham: British Association of Social Workers.

Baumann, S. (2021). L. Innovative communities: A global nursing perspective. *Nursing Science Quarterly*. 34(3), 316–321.

Baxter, K., Wilberforce, M. and Birks, Y. (2020). What skills do older self-funders in England need to arrange and manage social care? Findings from a scoping review of the literature. *The British Journal of Social Work*. bcaa102. https://doi.org/10.1093/bjsw/bcaa102.

BBC (2010). *Cameron and Clegg Set Out 'Big Society' Policy Ideas*. Retrieved from: www.news.bbc.co.uk/1/hi/uk_politics/8688860.stm.

Beard, R., Knauss, R. and Moyer, D. (2009). Managing disability and enjoying life: How we reframe dementia through personal narratives. *Journal of Aging Studies*. (23), 227–235.

Behuniak, S. (2011). The living dead? The construction of people with Alzheimer's disease as zombies. *Ageing & Society*. 31, 70–92.

Benbow, S. and Jolley, D. (2012). Dementia: Stigma and its effects. *Neurodegenerative Disease Management*. 2(2), 165–172.

Birt, L., Poland, F., Csipke, E. and Charlesworth, G. (2017). Shifting dementia discourses from deficit to active citizenship. *Sociology of Health & Illness*. 39(2), 199–211.

Blandin, K. and Pepin, R. (2017). Dementia grief: A theoretical model of a unique grief experience. *Dementia*. 16(1), 67–78.

Boise, L. (2014). Ethnicity and dementia. In Downs, M. and Bowers, B. (Eds). *Excellence in Dementia Care. Research into Practice* (2nd edition). Maidenhead: Open University Press. 36–52.

Bosco, A., Schneider, J., Coleston-Shields, D. M. and Orrell, M. (2019). Dementia care model: Promoting personhood through co-production. *Archives of Gerontology and Geriatrics*. 81, 59–73.

Boss, P. and Yeats, J. (2014). Ambiguous loss: A complicated type of grief when loved ones disappear. *Bereavement Care*. 33(2), 63–69.

Botsford, J. (2015). Communication and working with interpreters. In Botsford, J. and Harrison Dening, K. (Eds). *Dementia, Culture and Ethnicity, Issues for All*. London: Jessica Kingsley Publishers. 141–162.

Botsford, J. and Harrison Dening, K. (Eds). (2015). *Dementia, Culture and Ethnicity, Issues for All*. London: Jessica Kingsley Publishers.

Bowell, S. and Bamford, S. (2018). *What Would Life Be – Without a Song or Dance, What Are We?* London: The International Longevity Centre with the Utley Foundation.

Bradford Dementia Group (2005). *DCM 8 User's Manual*. Bradford: University of Bradford.

Brannelly, T. (2011). Sustaining citizenship: People with dementia and the phenomenon of social death. *Nursing Ethics*. 18(5), 662–671.

Braye, S. and Preston-Shoot, M. (Eds). (2020). *The Care Act 2014: Wellbeing in Practice*. London: Sage.

British Heart Foundation (2018). *Understanding Vascular Dementia*. Retrieved from: www.bhf.org.uk/informationsupport/publications/heart-conditions/vascular-dementia-quick-guide.

British Institute of Human Rights (2016a). *Dementia and Human Rights: A Practitioner's Guide*. London: The British Institute of Human Rights.

British Institute of Human Rights (2016b). *Social Care Intervention and Human Rights: A Practitioner's Guide*. London: The British Institute of Human Rights.

Brooker, D. (2004). What is person-centred care in dementia? *Reviews in Clinical Gerontology*. 13, 215–222.

Brooker, D. (2005). Dementia care mapping: A review of the research literature. *The Gerontologist*. 45 Special issue. 1(1), 11–18.

Brooker, D. (2007). *Person-Centred Dementia Care. Making Services Better*. London: Jessica Kingsley Publishers.

Brooker, D. and Latham, I. (2016). *Person-Centred Dementia Care. Making Services Better with the VIPS Framework* (2nd edition). London: Jessica Kingsley Publishers.

Brown, J., Huntley, D., Morgan, M., Dodson, K. and Cich, J. (2017). Confabulation: A guide for mental health professionals. *International Journal of Neurology and Neurotherapy*. 4(2), 1–9.

Buber, M. (1937). *Ich and Du (I and Thou)* (Translated by R. Gregor Smith). Edinburgh: Clark.

Buckner, L. and Yeandle, S. (2015). *Valuing Carers 2015*. London: Carers UK.

Butchard, S. and Kinderman, P. (2019). Human rights, dementia, and identity. *European Psychologist*. 24(2), 159–168.

Bywaters, P. (2007). Understanding the life course. In Lymbery, M. and Postle, K. (Eds). *Social Work: A Companion to Learning*. London: Sage. 134–144.

Cahill, S. (2020). WHO's global action plan on the public health response to dementia: Some challenges and opportunities. *Aging & Mental Health*. 24(2), 197–199.

Care Quality Commission (CQC) (2015). *Thinking About Using a Hidden Camera or Other Equipment to Monitor Someone's Care?* Retrieved from: https://narfire.org.uk/media/1196/cqc.pdf.

Care Quality Commission (CQC) (2016). *People with Dementia. A Different Ending: Addressing Inequalities in End of Life Care*. London: CQC.

Care Quality Commission (CQC) (2020a). *The State of Health Care and Adult Social Care in England 2019/20*, HC 799. London: CQC/HMSO.

Care Quality Commission (CQC) (2020b). *Technology in Care*. Retrieved from: www.cqc.org.uk/guidance-providers/all-services/technology-care.

carehome.co.uk (2021). *Care Home Fees and Costs:. How Much Do You Pay?* April 2021. Retrieved from: www.carehome.co.uk/advice/care-home-fees-and-costs-how-much-do-you-pay.

Carers UK (2012). *The Cost of Caring How Money Worries Are Pushing Carers to Breaking Point*. London: Carers UK.

Carling, C. (2012). *But Then Something Happened*. Cambridge: Golden Books.

Carr, S. (2010). *Personalisation: A Rough Guide* (revised edition). London: Social Care Institute for Excellence.

Cayton, H., Graham, N. and Warner, J. (2002). *Dementia. Alzheimer's and Other Dementias* (2nd edition). London: Class Publishing.

Cheston, R. and Bender, M. (1999). *Understanding Dementia. The Man with the Worried Eyes*. London: Jessica Kingsley Publishers.

Cheston, R. and Bradbury, N. (2018). *Evidence Briefing: Dementia, Accessibility and Minority Groups*. London: The British Psychological Society Dementia Advisory Group.

Clarke, C., Wilkinson, H., Keady, J. and Gibb, C. (2011). *Risk Assessment and Management for Living Well with Dementia*. London: Jessica Kingsley Publishers.

Community Care (2019). *How Personal Health Budgets in England Work: Key Information*. Retrieved from: www.communitycare.co.uk/2019/04/23/personal-health-budgets-england-work-key-information/.

Cooper, C., Selwood, A., Blanchard, M., Walker, Z., Blizard, R., Livingston, G. et al. (2009). Abuse of people with dementia by family carers: Representative cross sectional survey *BMJ*. 338, b155. doi:10.1136/bmj.b155.

Corner, J. (2017). Dementia is a terrible word. Why do people still use it? *The Guardian Newspaper*, 30 September 2017.

Coulshed, V. and Orme, J. (2012). *Social Work Practice*. Basingstoke: Palgrave.

Craig, C. (2004). Reaching out with the arts: Meeting with the person with dementia. In Innes, A., Archibald, C. and Murphy, C. (Eds). *Dementia and Social Inclusion*. London: Jessica Kingsley Publishers. 184–198.

Cutcliffe, J. and Herth, K. (2002). The concept of hope in nursing: Its origins, background and nature. *British Journal of Nursing*. 11(12), 832–840.

Davis, D. (2004). Dementia: Sociological and philosophical constructions. *Social Science & Medicine*. 58(2), 369–378.

De Vries, K. (2003). Palliative care for people with dementia. In Adams, T. and Manthorpe, J. (Eds). *Dementia Care*. London: Arnold. 114–135.

DEEP (2014). *Dementia Words Matter: Guidelines on Language About Dementia*. Exeter: Innovations in Dementia/The Dementia Engagement and Empowerment Project (DEEP).

Dementia Action Alliance (2015). *Words Matter: See Me Not My Dementia*. Retrieved from: daanow.org/wp-content/uploads/2016/03/Words_Matter-See-Me-Not-My-Dementia.pdf.

Dementia Alliance International (2019). *Supporting Dementia Self Advocates: A Directory of Resources*. Retrieved from: www.dementiaallianceinternational.org/wp-content/uploads/2019/07/Directory-of-Dementia-Self-Advocacy-Resources_July-2019_1st-Edition.pdf.

Dementia Australia (2018). *Dementia Language Guidelines*. Retrieved from: www.dementia.org.au/sites/default/files/full-language-guidelines.pdf.

Dementia Statistics (2021a). *Comorbidities*. Retrieved from: www.dementiastatistics.org/statistics/comorbidities/.

Dementia Statistics (2021b). *Different Types of Dementia*. Retrieved from: www.dementiastatistics.org/statistics/different-types-of-dementia/.

Dementia Statistics (2021c). *Prevalence by Gender in the UK*. Retrieved from: www.dementiastatistics.org/statistics/prevalence-by-gender-in-the-uk.

Dementia Statistics (2021d). *Memory Clinics*. Retrieved from: www.dementiastatistics.org/statistics/memory-clinics/.

Dementia UK (n.d. a). *Mixed Dementia*. Retrieved from: www.dementiauk.org/understanding-dementia/types-and-symptoms/mixed-dementia/?gclid=EAIaIQobChMItzO7c3V7wIVWuztCh3yPAvHEAAYASAAEgKUCfD_BwE.

Dementia UK (n.d. b). *What do Admiral Nurses Do?* Retrieved from: www.dementiauk.org/for-professionals/how-to-become-an-admiral-nurse/what-do-admiral-nurses-do/.

Dementia UK (2017). *A Template for Putting Together Life Story Books*. Retrieved from: www.dementiauk.org/life-story-work/.

Department for Constitutional Affairs (2007). *Mental Capacity Act 2005 Code of Practice*. London: TSO.

Department of Health (2005a). *The Mental Capacity Act*. London: HMSO.

Department of Health (2005b) *Building Telecare in England*. London: DH Publications.

Department of Health (2008). *End of Life Care Strategy Promoting High Quality Care for All Adults at the End of Life*. London: DH Publications.

Department of Health (2009). *The National Dementia Strategy: Living Well with Dementia*. London: DH Publications.

Department of Health (2010a). *Quality Outcomes for People with Dementia: Building on the Work of the National Dementia Strategy*. London: DH Publications.

Department of Health (2010b). *'Nothing Ventured, Nothing Gained': Risk Guidance for People with Dementia*. London: DH Publications.

Department of Health (2011a). *Living Well with Dementia: A National Dementia Strategy Good Practice Compendium – an Assets Approach*. London: DH Publications.

Department of Health (2011b). *Statement of Government Policy on Adult Safeguarding. Gateway Reference: 16072.* Retrieved from: https://assets.publishing.service.gov.uk/government/uploads/system/uploads/attachment_data/file/215591/dh_126770.pdf.

Department of Health (2012). *Prime Minister's Challenge on Dementia Delivering Major Improvements in Dementia Care and Research by 2015.* London: DH Publications.

Department of Health (2014). *Care and Support Statutory Guidance: Issued Under the Care Act 2014.* London: Department of Health. Most recent update 21 April 2021 Retrieved from: www.gov.uk/government/publications/care-act-statutory-guidance/care-and-support-statutory-guidance.

Department of Health (2015a). *Prime Minister's Challenge on Dementia 2020.* London: DH Publications.

Department of Health (2015b). *A Manual for Good Social Work Practice Supporting Adults Who Have Dementia.* London: DH Publications.

Department of Health (2015c). *Knowledge and Skills Statement for Social Workers in Adult Services.* Retrieved from: https://assets.publishing.service.gov.uk/government/uploads/system/uploads/attachment_data/file/411957/KSS.pdf.

Department of Health (2016). *Prime Minister's Challenge on Dementia 2020 Implementation Plan.* London: DH Publications.

Department of Health and Social Care (2018a). *Carers Action Plan 2018–2020 Supporting Carers Today.* London: Department of Health and Social Care.

Department of Health and Social Care (2018b). *National Framework for NHS Continuing Healthcare and NHS-funded Nursing Care.* October 2018 (Revised). London: Department of Health and Social Care.

Department of Health and Social Care (2018c). *Public Information Leaflet NHS Continuing Healthcare and NHS-Funded Nursing Care.* London: Department of Health and Social Care.

Department of Health and Social Care (2021). *Supporting People Living with Dementia to Be Involved in Adult Safeguarding Enquiries.* London: Department of Health and Social Care/University of Bath.

Dewing, J. (2008). Personhood and dementia: Revisiting Tom Kitwood's ideas. *International Journal of Older People Nursing.* 3(1), 3–13.

Dewing, J. and McCormack, B. (2016). Editorial: Tell me, how do you define person-centredness? *Journal of Clinical Nursing.* 26, 2509–2510.

Downs, M. (2000). Dementia in a socio-cultural context: An idea whose time has come. *Ageing and Society.* 20, 369–375.

Downs, M., Clare, L. and Mackenzie, J. (2006). Understandings of dementia: Explanatory models and their implications in Hughes, J., Louw, S. and Sabat, S. (Eds). *Dementia Mind, Meaning and the Person.* Oxford: Oxford University Press. 234–257.

Doyle, P. and Rubinstein, R. (2014). Person-centered dementia care and the cultural matrix of othering. *The Gerontologist.* 54(6), 952–963.

Elder, G. and Johnson, M. (2003). The life course and aging: Challenges, lessons, and new directions. In Settersten, R. and Hendricks, J. (Eds). *Invitation to the Life Course: Towards New Understandings of Later Life.* London: Routledge. 49–81.

Engel, G. (1977). The need for a new medical model: A challenge for biomedicine. *Science.* 196, 129–136.

Epps, D. and Furman, R. (2016). The 'alien other': A culture of dehumanizing immigrants in the United States. *Social Work & Society.* 14(2), 1–14.

Equality and Human Rights Commission (2011). *Close to Home: An Inquiry into Older People and Human Rights in Home Care.* London: Equality and Human Rights Commission.

Estes, C. and Binney, M. (1989). The biomedicalization of aging: Dangers and dilemmas. *The Gerontologist.* 29(5), 587–596.

Fage, B., Chan, C., Gill, S. S., Noel-Storr, A., Herrmann, N., Smailagic, N., Nikolaou, V. and Seitz, D. (2015). Mini-cog for the diagnosis of Alzheimer's disease dementia and other dementias within a community setting. *Cochrane Database of Systematic Reviews 2015* (2).

Fage, B., Chan, C., Gill, S. S., Noel-Storr, A., Herrmann, N., Smailagic, N., Nikolaou, V. and Seitz, D. (2019). Mini-Cog for the diagnosis of Alzheimer's disease dementia and other dementias within a secondary care setting. *Cochrane Database of Systematic Reviews*. 2019(9).

Fang, B. and Yan, E. (2018). Abuse of older persons with dementia: A review of the literature. *Trauma, Violence, & Abuse*. 19(2), 127–147.

Farre, A. and Rapley, T. (2017). The new old (and old new) medical model: Four decades navigating the biomedical and psychosocial understandings of health and illness. *Healthcare*. 5(4), 88.

Feil, N. (1993). *The Validation Breakthrough*. Cleveland: Health Professions Press.

Fiske, J. (2010). *Understanding Popular Culture* (2nd edition). London: Routledge.

Fletcher, J. (2019). Destigmatising dementia: The dangers of felt stigma and benevolent othering. *Dementia*. doi:10.1177/1471301219884821.

Fletcher, J. (2020). Mythical dementia and Alzheimerised senility: Discrepant and intersecting representations of cognitive decline in later life. *Social Theory & Health*. 18, 50–65.

Fossey, J. (2014). Care homes. In Downs, M. and Bowers, B. (Eds). *Excellence in Dementia Care. Research into Practice* (2nd edition). Maidenhead: Open University Press. 343–359.

Froggatt, K. and Goodman, C. (2014). Palliative care. In Downs, M. and Bowers, B. (Eds). *Excellence in Dementia Care. Research into Practice* (2nd edition). Maidenhead: Open University Press. 359–370.

G8 UK (2013). *G8 Dementia Summit Declaration*. Retrieved from: https://assets.publishing.service.gov.uk/government/uploads/system/uploads/attachment_data/file/265869/2901668_G8_DementiaSummitDeclaration_acc.pdf.

Gaylard, D. (2013). Assessing need. In Mantell, A. (Ed). *Skills for Social Work Practice* (2nd edition). London: Sage. 186–206.

George, D. and Whitehouse, P. (2014). The war (on terror) on Alzheimer's. *Dementia*. 13(1), 120–130.

Gibbons, J. and Plath, D. (2006). "Everybody puts a lot into it!" single session contacts in hospital social work. *Social Work in Health Care*. 42(1), 17–34.

Gilleard, C. and Higgs, P. (2010). Aging without agency: Theorizing the fourth age. *Aging and Mental Health*. 14(2), 121–128.

Gilleard, C. and Higgs, P. (2014). Studying dementia: The relevance of the fourth age. *Quality in Ageing: Policy, Practice and Research*. 15(4), 241–243.

Gilleard, C. and Higgs, P. (2015). Social death and the moral identity of the fourth age. *Journal of the Academy of Social Sciences*. 10(3), 1–10.

Gilliard, J., Means, R., Beattie, A. and Daker-White, G. (2005). Dementia care in England and the social model of disability: Lessons and issues. *Dementia*. 4(4), 571–586.

Global Council on Brain Health (2020). *The Brain-Heart Connection: GCBH Recommendations to Manage Cardiovascular Risks to Brain Health*. Washington, DC: Global Council on Brain Health.

Goffman, E. (1963). *Stigma: Notes on the Management of a Spoiled Identity*. New York: Simon & Schuster.

Goldman, J., Williams-Gray, C., Barker, R., Duda, J. and Galvin, J. (2014). The spectrum of cognitive impairment in Lewy body diseases. *Movement Disorders: Official Journal of the Movement Disorder Society*. 29(5), 608–621.

Goodorally, V. (2015). Access, assessment and engagement. In Botsford, J. and Harrison Dening, K. (Eds). *Dementia, Culture and Ethnicity, Issues for All*. London: Jessica Kingsley Publishers. 127–140.

Greenwood, D. (1998). Review of dementia reconsidered: The person comes first. *European Journal of Psychotherapy & Counselling.* 1 (1), 154–157.

Greenwood, N., Smith, R., Akhtar, F. and Richardson, A. (2017). A qualitative study of carers' experiences of dementia cafés: A place to feel supported and be yourself. *BMC Geriatrics.* 17(1), 164.1–9.

Gregory, M. and Holloway, M. (2005). Language and the shaping of social work. *British Journal of Social Work.* 35(1), 37–53.

Griffiths, A. W., Kelley, R., Garrod, L. et al. (2019). Barriers and facilitators to implementing dementia care mapping in care homes: Results from the DCM™ EPIC trial process evaluation. *BMC Geriatrics.* 19, 37.1–16.

Gubrium, J. (1986). The social preservation of mind: The Alzheimer's disease experience. *Symbolic Interaction* (9), 37–51.

Gubrium, J. (1987). Structuring and destructuring the course of illness: The Alzheimer's disease experience. *Sociology of Health & Illness* (9), 1–24.

Hampson, C. and Morris, K. (2016). Dementia: Sustaining self in the face of cognitive decline. *Geriatrics.* 1(4), 25.1–6.

Harding, N. and Palfrey, C. (1997). *The Social Construction of Dementia: Confused Professionals?* London: Jessica Kingsley Publishers.

Harrop, E., Morgan, F., Byrne, A. and Nelson, A. (2016). "It still haunts me whether we did the right thing": A qualitative analysis of free text survey data on the bereavement experiences and support needs of family caregivers. *BMC Palliative Care.* 15(92), 1–8.

Heenan, D. (2021). Hospital social work and discharge planning for older people: Challenges of working in a clinical setting. *Ageing and Society.* 1–18. doi:10.1017/S0144686X21001124.

Henderson, A. and World Health Organization. (1994). *Dementia.* Geneva: World Health Organization.

Henderson, K. and Mathew-Byrne, J. (2016). Developing communication and interviewing skills. In Davies, K. and Jones, R. (Eds). *Skills for Social Work Practice.* Basingstoke: Palgrave. 1–22.

Henwood, C. and Downs, M. (2014). Dementia-friendly communities. In Downs, M. and Bowers, B. (Eds). *Excellence in Dementia Care. Research into Practice* (2nd edition). Buckingham: Open University Press.

Higgs, P. and Gilleard, C. (2016). Interrogating personhood and dementia. *Aging & Mental Health.* 20(8), 773–780.

Hillman, A. and Latimer, J. (2017). Cultural representations of dementia. *PLoS Medicine.* 14(3), e1002274.

HM Government (2008). *Carers at the Heart of 21st-Century Families and Communities.* London: The Stationery Office.

HM Government (2010). *Recognised, Valued and Supported: Next Steps for the Carers Strategy.* London: The Stationery Office.

HM Government (2014). *The Care Act 2014.* London: The Stationery Office.

Holder, H., Kumpunen, S., Castle-Clarke, S. and Lombardo, S. (2018). *Managing the Hospital and Social Care Interface Interventions Targeting Older Adults.* London: The Nuffield Trust.

Holden, U. and Woods, R. (1988). *Reality Orientation: Psychological Approaches to the Confused Elderly.* Edinburgh: Churchill Livingstone.

Hood, R. (2016). Assessment for social work practice. In Davies, K. and Jones, R. (Eds). *Skills for Social Work Practice.* Basingstoke: Palgrave. 82–102.

Hospice UK (2015). *Hospice Enabled Dementia Care the First Steps.* London: Hospice UK.

Hughes, J. and Baldwin, C. (2006). *Ethical Issue in Dementia Care.* London: Jessica Kingsley Publishers.

Huppert, F., Brayne, C. and O'Connor, D. (1994). *Dementia and Normal Aging*. Cambridge: Cambridge University Press.

Hyden, L. (2011). Non-verbal vocalizations, dementia and social interaction. *Communication & Medicine*. 8(2), 135–144.

Innes, A. (2009). *Dementia Studies*. London: Sage.

Innes, A., Archibald, C. and Murphy, C. (2004). (Eds). *Dementia and Social Inclusion*. London: Jessica Kingsley Publishers.

Innes, A. and Manthorpe, J. (2012). Developing theoretical understandings of dementia and their application to dementia care policy in the UK. *Dementia*. 12(6), 682–696.

International Classification of Diseases (2016). *'Organic, Including Symptomatic, Mental Disorders(F00-F09)' ICD-10, Version 2016, F00*. Retrieved from: https://icd.who.int/browse10/2016/en#!/F00-F09.

Jakhar, J., Ambreen, S. and Prasad, S. (2021). Right to life or right to die in advanced dementia: Physician-assisted dying. *Frontiers in Psychiatry*. 11, 622446. doi:10.3389/fpsyt.2020.622446.

Jarvik, L., LaRue, A., Blacker, D., Gatz, M., Kawas, C., McArdle, J., Morris, J., Mortimer, J., Ringman, J., Ercoli, L., Freimer, N., Gokhman, I., Manly, J., Plassman, B., Rasgon, N., Roberts, J., Sunderland, T., Swan, G., Wolf, P. and Zonderman, A. (2008). Children of persons with Alzheimer disease: What does the future hold? *Alzheimer Disease and Associated Disorders*. 22(1), 6–20.

Jellinger, K. (2018). Dementia with Lewy bodies and Parkinson's disease-dementia: Current perspectives. *International Journal of Neurology and Neurotherapy*. 5(2), 1–11.

Joffe, H. (1999). *Risk and 'the Other'*. Cambridge: Cambridge University Press.

Johns, C. (1994). *The Burford NDU Model: Caring in Practice*. Oxford: Blackwell Science.

Joseph Rowntree Foundation (2012). *Creating a Dementia Friendly York*. Retrieved from: www.jrf.org.uk/sites/default/files/jrf/migrated/files/dementia-communities-york-summary.pdf.

Kadushin, A. and Kadushin, G. (2013). *The Social Work Interview* (5th edition). New York: Columbia University Press.

Khan, O. (2015). Dementia and ethnic diversity. In Botsford, J. and Harrison Dening, K. (Eds). *Dementia, Culture and Ethnicity, Issues for All*. London: Jessica Kingsley Publishers. 21–34.

Killick, J. and Allan, K. (2001). *Communication and the Care of People with Dementia*. Buckingham: Open University Press.

King's Fund (2006). *Direct Payments and Older People*. London: King's Fund.

King's Fund (2021). *The Social Care System Is Failing the People Who Rely on It and Urgently Needs Reform*. Retrieved from: www.kingsfund.org.uk/projects/positions/adult-social-care-funding-and-eligibility.

Kingston, A., Comas-Herrera, A. and Jagger, C. (2018). Forecasting the care needs of the older population in England over the next 20 years: Estimates from the population ageing and care simulation (PACSim) modelling study. *Lancet Public Health*. 3(9), 447–455.

Kitching, D. (2015). Depression in dementia. *Australian Prescriber*. 38(6), 209–211.

Kitwood, T. (1997). *Dementia Reconsidered: The Person Comes First*. Maidenhead: Open University Press.

Kitwood, T. and Bredin, K. (1992). Towards a theory of dementia care: Personhood and well-being. *Ageing and Society*. 12(3), 269–287.

Kitwood, T. and Brooker, D. (Eds). (2019). *Dementia Reconsidered, Revisited: The Person Still Comes First*. London: Open University Press.

Konigsberg, R. (2011). *The Truth About Grief: The Myth of Its Five Stages and the New Science of Loss*. New York: Simon & Schuster.

Kontos, P. (2005). Embodied selfhood in Alzheimer's disease. *Dementia*. 4, 553–570.

Kübler-Ross, E. (1989). *On Death and Dying*. London: Routledge.

Kwon, O. Y., Ahn, H. S., Kim, H. J. and Park, K. W. (2017). Effectiveness of cognitive behavioral therapy for caregivers of people with dementia: A systematic review and meta-analysis. *Journal of Clinical Neurology*. 13(4), 394–404.

Lakey, L. and Saunders, T. (2014). *Getting Personal? Making Personal Budgets Work*. London: Alzheimer's Society.

Lancet Neurology (2018). Response to the growing dementia burden must be faster. *Lancet Neurology (Editorial)*. 17(8), 651–651.

Lane, H., McLachlan, S. and Philip, J. (2013). The war against dementia: Are we battle weary yet? *Age and Ageing*. 42(3), 281–283.

Lane, P., Spencer, S., Smith, D. M., McCready, M., Roddam, M., Codona, J. and Barrett, S. (2021). *Saying It as It Is: Experiences of Gypsies and Travellers Caring for Family Members Living with Dementia*. Project Report. Cambridge: Anglia Ruskin University.

Lariviere, M., Poland, F., Woolham, J., Newman, S. and Fox, C. (2021). Placing assistive technology and telecare in everyday practices of people with dementia and their caregivers: Findings from an embedded ethnography of a national dementia trial. *BMC Geriatrics*. 21, 121.1–13.

Laslett, P. (1987). The emergence of the third age. *Ageing and Society*. 7, 133–160.

LGA (2014). *Making Safeguarding Personal: Guide 2014*. London: Local Government Association and ADASS.

LGA (2018). *Supporting Carers: Guidance and Case Studies*. London: Local Government Association.

LGA (2021). *Prevention*. Retrieved from: www.local.gov.uk/our-support/our-improvement-offer/care-and-health-improvement/integration-and-better-care-fund/better-care-fund/integration-resource-library/prevention.

Lishman, J. (2009). *Communication in Social Work* (2nd edition). Basingstoke: Palgrave.

Low, L-F. and Purwaningrum, F. (2020). Negative stereotypes, fear and social distance: A systematic review of depictions of dementia in popular culture in the context of stigma. *BMC Geriatrics*. 20, 477.

Lucas, S. (2020). *Spoken Language Interpreters in Social Work*. Retrieved from: www.iriss.org.uk/sites/default/files/2020-04/insights-52.pdf.

Luengo-Fernandez, R., Leal, J. and Gray, A. (2010). *Dementia 2010*. Cambridge: Alzheimer's Research Trust.

Lyman, K. (1989). Bringing the social back in: A critique of the biomedicalization of dementia. *The Gerontologist*. 29(5), 597–605.

MacIntyre, G., Stewart, A. and McCusker, P. (2018). *Safeguarding Adults*. Basingstoke: Palgrave.

MacRae, H. (2009). Managing identity while living with Alzheimer's disease. *Qualitative Health Research*. 20(3), 293–305.

Maffioletti, V., Baptista, M., Santos, R. L., Rodrigues, V. M. and Dourado, M. (2019). Effectiveness of day care in supporting family caregivers of people with dementia: A systematic review. *Dementia & Neuropsychologia*. 13(3), 268–283.

Mantell, A. and Scragg, T. (Eds). (2019). *Reflective Practice in Social Work* (5th edition). London: Learning Matters.

Manthorpe, J. (2004). Risk taking. In Innes, A., Archibald, C. and Murphy, C. (Eds). *Dementia and Social Inclusion*. London: Jessica Kingsley Publishers. 137–152.

Marie Curie (2015). *The Hidden Costs of Caring*. London: Marie Curie.

Mayrhofer, A., Mathie, E., McKeown, J., Bunn, F. and Goodman, C. (2018). Age-appropriate services for people diagnosed with young onset dementia (YOD): A systematic review. *Aging & Mental Health*. August; 22(8), 927–935.

McColgan, G. (2004). Images, constructs, theory and method: Including the narrative of dementia. In Innes, A., Archibald, C. and Murphy, C. (Eds). *Dementia and Social Inclusion*. London: Jessica Kingsley Publishers. 169–183.

McCormack, B. (2004). Person-centredness in gerontological nursing: An overview of the literature. *Journal of Clinical Nursing*. 13(3A), 31–38.

McCurry, S., Reynolds, C., Ancoli-Israel, S., Teri, L. and Vitiello, M. (2000). Treatment of sleep disturbance in Alzheimer's disease. *Sleep Medicine Reviews*. 4(6), 603–628.

McGovern, J. (2015). Living better with dementia: Strengths-based social work practice and dementia care. *Social Work in Health Care*. 54(5), 408–421.

Mental Health Foundation (2015). *Dementia, Rights, and the Social Model of Disability a New Direction for Policy and Practice?* London: The Mental Health Foundation.

Milne, A. and Smith, J. (2015). Dementia, ethnicity and care homes. In Botsford, J. and Harrison Dening, K. (Eds). *Dementia, Culture and Ethnicity, Issues for All*. London: Jessica Kingsley Publishers. 197–218.

Moriarty, J. and Manthorpe, J. (2016). *The Effectiveness of Social Work with Adults: A Systematic Scoping Review*. London: King's College. Retrieved from: https://www.kcl.ac.uk/sspp/policy-institute/scwru/pubs/2016/reports/Moriarty-&- Manthorpe-2016-Effectiveness-of-social-work-with-adults.pdf.

Morrison, T. (2006). Emotional intelligence, emotion and social work: Context, characteristics, complications and contribution. *British Journal of Social Work*. 37(2), 245–263.

Mukadam, N., Cooper, C. and Livingston, G. (2013). Improving access to dementia services for people from minority ethnic groups. *Current Opinion in Psychiatry*. 26(4), 409–414.

Munby, J. (2007). The case of Local Authority X v MM & Another (No 1) (2007). Retrieved from: https://www.familylawweek.co.uk/site.aspx?i=ed863

NAO (2017). *Investigation into NHS Continuing Healthcare Funding*. HC 239. London: National Audit Office/Department of Health and Social Care.

National Audit Office (2021). *The Adult Social Care Market in England*. London: National Audit Office/ Department of Health & Social Care.

Nelson-Becker, H., Lloyd, L., Milne, A., Perry, E., Ray, M., Richards, S., Sullivan, M., Tanner, D. and Willis, P. (2020). Strengths-based social work with older people: A UK perspective. In *Rooted in Strengths: Celebrating the Strengths Perspective in Social Work*. Kansas: University of Kansas Libraries. 327–346.

Newbronner, L., Chamberlain, R., Borthwick, R., Baxter, M. and Glendinning, C. (2013). *A Road Less Rocky – Supporting People with Dementia*. London: Carers Trust.

NHS (2021). *Alzheimer's Disease*. Retrieved from: www.nhs.uk/conditions/alzheimers-disease/.

NHS (n.d.). *About Dementia*. Retrieved from: www.nhs.uk/conditions/dementia/about.

NHS England (2014). *NHS England's Commitment to Carers*. Leeds: NHS England.

NHS England (2018). *My Future Wishes. Advance Care Planning (ACP) for People with Dementia in All Care Settings*. Leeds: NHS England.

NHS England (2021). *Dementia*. Retrieved from: www.england.nhs.uk/mental-health/dementia/.

NICE (2018). *Dementia: Assessment, Management and Support for People Living with Dementia and Their Carers*. Retrieved from: www.nice.org.uk/guidance/ng97/chapter/Recommendations.

NICE (n.d.). *Polypharmacy*. Retrieved from: www.rpharms.com/recognition/setting-professional-standards/polypharmacy.

NICE (2021). *Palliative Care – General Issues*. Retrieved from: cks.nice.org.uk/topics/palliative-care-general-issues/.

Nolan, M., Davies, S. and Grant, G. (2001). Integrating perspectives. In Nolan, M., Davies, S. and Grant, G. (Eds). *Working with Older People and Their Families: Key Issues in Policy and Practice*. Buckingham: Open University Press. 160–178.

Norris, A. (1986). *Reminiscence with Elderly People*. London: Winslow.

Ogden, J. (2017). Rising cost of dementia care risks social care funding crisis. *Progress in Neurology and Psychiatry*. 21(1), 5.

O'Loughlin, M. and O'Loughlin, S. (Eds). (2015). *Effective Observation in Social Work Practice*. London: Sage.

Packer, T. (2003). Turning rhetoric into reality: Person-centred approaches for community mental health nursing. In Keady, J., Clarke, C. and Adams, T. (Eds). *Community Mental Health Nursing and Dementia Care*. Maidenhead: Open University Press. 104–119.

Parker, J. (2001). Interrogating person centred dementia care in social work and social care practice. *Journal of Social Work*. 1(3), 329–345.

Pattoni, L. (2012). *Strengths-Based Approaches for Working with Individuals*. Glasgow: Iriss. Retrieved from: iriss.org.uk/resources/insights/strengths-based-approaches-working-individuals.

Parker, J. (2003). Positive communication with people who have dementia. In Adams, T. and Manthorpe, J. (Eds). *Dementia Care*. London: Arnold. 148–163.

Parsons, C. (2017). Polypharmacy and inappropriate medication use in patients with dementia: An under researched problem. *Therapeutic Advances in Drug Safety*. 8(1), 31–46.

Peel, E. (2014). 'The living death of Alzheimer's' versus 'Take a walk to keep dementia at bay': Representations of dementia in print media and carer discourse. *Sociology of Health & Illness*. 36(6).

Phillipson, L., Hall, D., Cridland, E., Fleming, R., Brennan-Horley, C., Guggisberg, N., Frost, D. and Hasan, H. (2019). Involvement of people with dementia in raising awareness and changing attitudes in a dementia friendly community pilot project. *Dementia*. 18(7–8), 2679–2694.

Porter, R. (2003). *Madness: A Brief History*. Oxford: Oxford University Press.

Post, S. (2000). *The Moral Challenge of Alzheimer's Disease* (2nd edition). London: The John Hopkins University Press.

Prince, M., Knapp, M., Guerchet, M., McCrone, P., Prina, M., Comas-Herrera, M., Wittenberg, A., Adelaja, R., Hu, B., King, B., Rehill, D. and Salimkumar, D. (2014). *Dementia UK: Update*. London: Alzheimer's Society.

Public Health England (2019a). *Dementia: Comorbidities in Patients – Data Briefing*. Retrieved from: www.gov.uk/government/publications/dementia-comorbidities-in-patients/dementia-comorbidities-in-patients-data-briefing.

Public Health England (2019b). *Statistical Commentary: Dementia Profile, April 2019 Update*. Retrieved from: www.gov.uk/government/statistics/dementia-profile-april-2019-data-update/statistical-commentary-dementia-profile-april-2019-update.

Rare Dementia Support Group (2022). *What Is Rare Dementia?* Retrieved from: www.raredementiasupport.org/what-is-rare-dementia.

Ravalier, J. and Boichat, C. (2018). *UK Social Workers: Working Conditions and Wellbeing (August 2018)*. Bath: Bath Spa University.

Reilly, J. and Houghton, C. (2019). The experiences and perceptions of care in acute settings for patients living with dementia: A qualitative evidence synthesis. *International Journal of Nursing Studies*, 82–90.

Richards, C. (Ed). (2020). *Living Well with Dementia Through Music*. London: Jessica Kingsley Publishers.

Rimmer, L. (1982). *Reality Orientation: Principles and Practice*. London: Winslow.

Rizzi, L., Rosset, I. and Roriz-Cruz, M. (2014). Global epidemiology of dementia: Alzheimer's and vascular types. *BioMed Research International*. 2014, 908915.

Robinson, L., Dickinson, C., Bamford, C., Clark, A., Hughes, J. and Exley, C. (2013). A qualitative study: Professionals' experiences of advance care planning in dementia and palliative care, 'a good idea in theory but. . .' *Palliative Medicine*. 27(5), 401–408.

Rogers, C. (1961). *On Becoming a Person*. Boston: Houghton Mifflin Co.

Røsvik, J., Kirkevold, M., Engedal, K., Kirkevoldand, Ø. and Brooker, D. (2011). A model for using the VIPS framework for person-centred care for persons with dementia in nursing homes: A qualitative evaluative study. *International Journal of Older People Nursing*. 6(3), 227–236.

Sabat, S. (2001). *The Experience of Alzheimer's Disease – Life Through a Tangled Veil*. Oxford: Blackwell.

Sabat, S. (2014). A bio-psycho-social approach to dementia. In Downs, M. and Bowers, B. (Eds). *Excellence in Dementia Care. Research into Practice* (2nd edition). Maidenhead: Open University Press. 107–121.

Sabat, S. and Harré, R. (1992). The construction and deconstruction of self in Alzheimer's disease. *Ageing and Society*. 12, 443–461.

Saleeby, D. (1996). The strengths perspective in social work practice Extensions and cautions. *Social Work*. 41(3), 296–305.

Schölin, L., Rhynas, S., Holloway, A. and Jepson, R. (2019). *Rapid Evidence Review Dual Diagnosis, Double Stigma: A Rapid Review of Experiences of Living with Alcohol-Related Brain Damage (ARBD)*. London: Alcohol Change UK.

SCIE (n.d.). *Dementia at a Glance*. Retrieved from: www.scie.org.uk/dementia/about/

SCIE (2010). *Personalisation Briefing. Implications for Social Workers in Adults' Services*. London: Social Care Institute for Excellence.

SCIE (2012). *Protecting Adults at Risk: Good Practice Guide*. London: Social Care Institute for Excellence.

SCIE (2013). *Co-Production in Social Care: What It Is and How to Do It*. Retrieved from: www.scie.org.uk/publications/guides/guide51/what-is-coproduction/defining-copro duction.asp.

SCIE (2015). *Care Act 2014 Assessment and Eligibility Process Map*. Retrieved from: www. scie.org.uk/care-act-2014/assessment-and-eligibility/process-map/.

SCIE (2020). *End-of-Life Care and Dementia: An Introduction*. Retrieved from: www.scie. org.uk/dementia/advanced-dementia-and-end-of-life-care/end-of-life-care/introduc tion.asp.

Scourfield, P. (2015). Implementing co-production in adult social care: An example of meta-governance failure? *Social Policy and Society*. 14(4), 541–554.

Scourfield, P. (2021). *Using Advocacy in Social Work Practice*. London: Routledge.

Scrutton, J. and Barancati, C. (2016). *Dementia and Comorbidities: Ensuring Parity of Care*. London: International Longevity Centre UK.

Settersten, R. and Hendricks, J. (Eds). (2003). *Invitation to the Life Course: Towards New Understandings of Later Life*. London: Routledge.

Shakespeare, T. (2006). *Disability Rights and Wrongs*. London: Routledge.

Shakespeare, T., Zeilig, H. and Mittler, P. (2019). Rights in mind: Thinking differently about dementia and disability. *Dementia*. 18(3), 1075–1088.

Shannon, K., Bail, K. and Neville, S. (2019). Dementia-friendly community initiatives: An integrative review. *Journal of Clinical Nursing*. 28(11–12), 2035–2045.

Shön, D. (1983). *The Reflective Practitioner*. New York: Basic Books.

Shulman, L. (2008). *The Skills of Helping Individuals Families, Groups and Communities* (6th edition). Belmont, CA: Brooks/Cole.

Skills for Care (2015/2018). *Dementia Core Skills Education and Training Framework*. London: Skills for Care, Skills for Health and Health Education England.

Skills for Care (2020). *The State of the Adult Social Care Sector and Workforce in England*. Leeds: Skills for Care.

Smethurst, C., Robson, J. and Killner, V. (2013). Skills in working with risk. In Mantell, A. (Ed). *Skills for Social Work Practice* (2nd edition). London: Sage. 207–225.

Smith, T. (2004). *Living with Alzheimer's Disease* (2nd edition). London: Sheldon Press.

Social Work England (2019). *Professional Standards Guidance*. Sheffield: Social Work England.

Spector, A., Woods, B. and Orrell, M. (2008). Cognitive stimulation for the treatment of Alzheimer's disease. *Expert Review of Neurotherapeutics*. 8(5), 751–757.

Stanley, T. (2016). A practice framework to support the care act 2014. *The Journal of Adult Protection*. 18(1), 53–64.

Stephan, B. and Brayne, C. (2014). Prevalence and projections of dementia. In Downs, M. and Bowers, B. (Eds). *Excellence in Dementia Care. Research into Practice* (2nd edition). Maidenhead: Open University Press. 3–19.

Stokes, G. (2000). *Challenging Behaviour in Dementia. A Person-Centred Approach*. Bicester: Speechmark.

Stokes, G. and Goudie, F. (1990). *Working with Dementia*. Bicester: Winslow Press.

Stroebe, M. and Schut, H. (1999). The dual process model of coping with bereavement: Rationale and description. *Death Studies*. 23(3), 197–224.

Surr, C., Holloway, I., Walwyn, R., Griffiths, A., Meads, D., Martin, A., Kelley, R., Ballard, C., Fossey, J., Burnley, N., Chenoweth, L., Creese, B., Downs, M., Garrod, L., Graham, E., Lilley-Kelly, A., McDermid, J., McLellan, V., Millard, H., Perfect, D., Robinson, L., Robinson, O., Shoesmith, E., Siddiqi, N., Stokes, G., Wallace, D. and Farrin, J. (2020). Effectiveness of dementia care mapping™ to reduce agitation in care home residents with dementia: An open-cohort cluster randomised controlled trial. *Aging & Mental Health*, 1–14. https://doi.org/10.1080/13607863.2020.1745144.

Swaffer, K. (2014). Dementia: Stigma, language, and dementia-friendly. *Dementia*. 13(6), 709–716.

Sweeting, H. and Gilhooly, M. (1997). Dementia and the phenomenon of social death. *Sociology of Health & Illness*. 19(1), 93–117.

Symonds, J., Miles, C., Steel, M., Porter, S. and Williams, V. (2020). Making person-centred assessments. *Journal of Social Work*. 20(4), 431–447.

Teater, B. (2014). *Applying Social Work Theories and Methods* (2nd edition). Maidenhead: Open University press.

Teo, T. (Ed). (2014). *Encyclopedia of Critical Psychology*. New York: Springer.

Thompson, R. (2011). Using life story work to enhance care. *Nursing Older People*. 23(8), 16–21.

Thompson, S. and Thompson, N. (2018). *The Critically Reflective Practitioner* (2nd edition). Basingstoke: Palgrave MacMillan.

Titchen, A. (2001). Skilled companionship in professional practice. In Higgs, J. and Titchen, A. (Eds). *Practice Knowledge and Expertise in the Health Professions*. Oxford: Butterworth Heinemann. 69–79.

Titterton, M. (2005). *Risk and Risk Taking and Social Welfare*. London: Jessica Kingsley Publishers.

Tomlinson, E. and Stott, J. (2015). Assisted dying in dementia: A systematic review of the international literature on the attitudes of health professionals, patients, carers and the public, and the factors associated with these. *International Journal of Geriatric Psychiatry*. 30(1), 10–20.

Trang, N. and Xiaoming, L. (2020). Understanding public-stigma and self-stigma in the context of dementia: A systematic review of the global literature. *Dementia*. 19(2), 148–181.

Trevithick, P. (2012). *Social Work Skills and Knowledge a Practice Handbook* (3rd edition). Maidenhead: Open University Press.

Twigg, J. and Atkin, K. (1994). *Carers Perceived: Policy and Practice in Informal Care*. Buckingham: Open University Press.

UNCRPD (2006). UN General Assembly, Convention on the Rights of Persons with Disabilities: resolution/adopted by the General Assembly, 24 January 2007. Retrieved from: https://www.un.org/development/desa/disabilities/convention-on-the-rights-of-persons-with-disabilities.html.

Vermeer, Y., Higgs, P. and Charlesworth, G. (2019). What do we require from surveillance technology? A review of the needs of people with dementia and informal caregivers. *Journal of Rehabilitation and Assistive Technologies Engineering*. 6, 1–12.

Vernooij-Dassen, M., Moniz-Cook, E., Verhey, F., Chattat, R., Woods, B., Meiland, F., Franco, M., Holmerova, I., Orrell, M. and de Vugt, M. (2021). Bridging the divide between biomedical and psychosocial approaches in dementia research: The 2019 INTERDEM manifesto. *Aging & Mental Health*. 25(2), 206–212.

Whitlach, C. (2014). Understanding and enhancing the relationship between people with dementia and their family carers. In Downs, M. and Bowers, B. (Eds). *Excellence in Dementia Care. Research into Practice* (2nd edition). Maidenhead: Open University Press. 161–175.

Winblad, B., Amouyel, P., Andrieu, S., Ballard, C., Brayne, C., Brodaty, H., Cedazo-Minguez, A., Dubois, B., Edvardsson, D., Feldman, H., Fratiglioni, L., Frisoni, G., Gauthier, S., Georges, J., Graff, C., Iqbal, K., Jessen, F., Johansson, G., Jönsson, L., Kivipelto, M., Knapp, M., Mangialasche, F., Melis, R., Nordberg, A., Rikkert, M., Qiu, C., Sakmar, T., Scheltens, P., Schneider, L., Sperling, R., Tjernberg, L., Waldemar, G., Wimo, A. and Zetterberg, H. (2016). Defeating Alzheimer's disease and other dementias: A priority for European science and society. *Lancet Neurology*. 15(5), 455–532.

Wittenberg, R., Hu, B., Barraza-Araiza, L. and Rehill, A. (2019). *Projections of Older People with Dementia and Costs of Dementia Care in the United Kingdom, 2019–2040*. London: Care Policy and Evaluation Centre, London School of Economics and Political Science.

Woodhead, H. (2021). Film's struggle to help us understand the pain of dementia. *BBC Culture*. Retrieved from: www.bbc.com/culture/article/20210224-can-film-really-help-us-understand-the-pain-of-dementia.

Woods, B. (1999). Editorial: The legacy of Kitwood: Professor Tom Kitwood 1937–1998. *Aging & Mental Health*. 3(1), 5–7.

Woods, B., O'Philbin, L., Farrell, E. M., Spector, A. E. and Orrell, M. (2018). Reminiscence therapy for dementia. *The Cochrane Database of Systematic Reviews*. 3(3).

World Health Organisation (2004). *Ageing and Health Technical Report, Volume 5: A Glossary of Terms for Community Health Care and Services for Older Persons*. Geneva: World Health Organization.

World Health Organization (2012). *Dementia: A Public Health Priority*. Geneva: World Health Organization.

World Health Organization (2015a). *First WHO Ministerial Conference on Global Action Against Dementia*. Geneva: World Health Organization.

World Health Organization (2015b). *Ensuring a Human Rights-Based Approach for People Living with Dementia*. Geneva: World Health Organization.

World Health Organisation (2017). *WHO Global Action Plan on the Public Health Response to Dementia 2017–25*. Geneva: World Health Organization.

World Health Organization (2020). *Dementia*. Retrieved from: www.who.int/news-room/fact-sheets/detail/dementia.

Zarit, H. and Zarit, J. (2014). Supporting families coping with dementia: Flexibility and change. In Downs, M. and Bowers, B. (Eds). *Excellence in Dementia Care. Research into Practice* (2nd edition). Maidenhead: Open University Press. 176–187.

Zeilig, H. (2013). Dementia as a cultural metaphor. *The Gerontologist.* 54(2), 258–267.

Zeilig, H. (2014). Representations of people with dementia in the media and in literature. In Downs, M. and Bowers, B. (Eds). *Excellence in Dementia Care. Research into Practice* (2nd edition). Maidenhead: Open University Press. 70–91.

# INDEX

Note: Page numbers in *italics* indicate a figure on the corresponding page.

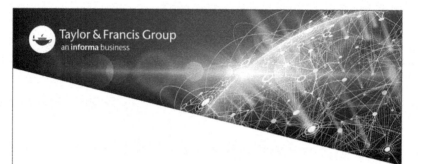